Mathematics for Healthcare Professionals

Mathematics for Healthcare Professionals

A Text/Workbook with Applications

Edward M. Stumpf

Frederick R. Fritz

William W. Bradford
Central Carolina Community College

Carolina Academic Press
Durham, NC

ISBN 10: 1-59460-320-0
ISBN 13: 978-1-59460-320-4
LCCN 2007930149

Carolina Academic Press
700 Kent Street
Durham, NC 27701
Telephone (919) 489-7486
Fax (919) 493-5668
www.cap-press.com

Printed in the United States of America

Contents

Introduction

This text provides a one-semester course in the basics of mathematics needed for Healthcare Professionals such as nursing students, medical assistants and technicians and dental hygienists and assistants. The course covers fractions, decimals and percentage without the use of calculators as is the case on many State Board Exams. The language is designed to be readable and in terms of everyday usage rather than formal and strict mathematical terms.

In addition to basic mathematical computations, several chapters are devoted to application problems involving dosage, concentration and dilution of solutions. The English and Metric systems of measurement are included with intra– and inter–system conversion and computation. An introduction to reading graphs is presented as well as a chapter on basic statistical concepts and using basic statistical measures. A chapter on algebra is included.

The workbook style of the text allows students freedom to move at a pace that ensures mastery of the material as well as flexibility for covering topics in any prescribed manner. Students should read the material, study the examples, and work all the exercises in a particular problem set before checking answers. The answers to odd–numbered exercises are provided in the Answer Keys.

In many programs, this may be the only math course students are required to take. If this is one of your early course offerings, the material will be valuable and useful in other courses, in particular chemistry and clinical practices labs.

The intent and focus of this text is on practical mathematical techniques and concepts. It is NOT intended as a course on medications or the administration of medications. Any medicine references in the text are used to illustrate and practice arithmetic, and may not be the actual dosages or concentrations available or used.

It is our hope that you will find the material useful and pertinent. If you have comments or suggestions please contact me at:

Edward Stumpf
Central Carolina Community College
estumpf@cccc.edu

Unit I

Chapter 1
Roman Numerals

Two systems of numeration are used by physicians and technicians – Arabic Numerals and Roman Numerals. The Arabic system utilizes the numerals 0, 1, 2, 3, 4, 5, 6, 7, 8, 9. It is the system most commonly used in all fields. All numerical values may be expressed by combinations of these ten symbols. The Arabic system is used to express weights and measures of the metric system and fractional units of the apothecaries' system.

The Roman system is sometimes used to indicate small quantities as well as being used in prescriptions. Roman numerals are encountered less often these days than in the past. Still, some knowledge of Roman numerals is desired of the technician. There are several simple rules governing Roman numerals.

Various Roman numerals in common use are:

Arabic	Roman
1	I or i
5	V or v
10	X or x
50	L or l
100	C
500	D
1000	M

In the Roman system, seven letters are used as symbols for numerals (indicated above). These letters are combined to express numerical values. When the apothecary system of measurement is used, whole units are expressed by Roman numerals. Lowercase or uppercase (capital) letters may be used to express Roman numerals, but it is customary to use small letters to indicate values of apothecary units. Cases are not mixed. Values over 30 are seldom used in medical practice. However, Roman numerals above 30 are encountered occasionally and the medical practitioner should be familiar with the rules governing their use. The lower-case Roman numeral i (1) is always written with a dot over it to avoid confusion with the lower-case Roman letter l (50). In modern times, the use of lowercase Roman numerals has declined for values of fifty or more, but are used more extensively for lesser values.

When reading or writing Roman numerals, pay attention to the position of the lesser values of numerals, such as I or V, in relation to the numerals of greater value, such as X or L.

Rules for Reading or Writing Roman Numerals

1) When a numeral is followed by the same numeral or by one of lesser value, the values of the numerals are added:

ii or II	xiii or XIII	xv or XV
means 1 + 1 or 2	means 10 + 1 + 1 + 1 or 13	means 10 + 5 or 15

2) When a numeral is written before one of greater value, the lesser value is subtracted from the greater one.

iv or IV	ix or IX
means 5 – 1 or 4	means 10 – 1 or 9

3) When a numeral is written between two or more numerals of greater value, its value is subtracted from the sum of the others in the numeral.

xix or XIX	xxxix or XXXIX
means 10 + 10 – 1 = 20 – 1 or 19	means 10 + 10 + 10 + 10 – 1 = 40 – 1 or 39

xxiv or XXIV	XLIX
10 + 10 + 5 –1 = 24	50 – 10 + 10 – 1 = 49

4)   A single one, I (i) can precede only V (v) or X (x)

iv = 4 or IX = 9 are okay

IIX or IIL or IL are *not* okay.

A single X (x) can precede only L or C .

XL for 40   or   XC for 90

A single value for 100, C, can precede only D or M

CD = 400   CM = 900   CDXC = 490

5)   The numerals I (i), X (x), C and M are used a maximum of three times in succession. The numerals for 5 and 50, V (v) and L, respectively, are never used in succession.

iii or III   xxx or XXX

means 1 + 1 + 1 is 3   means 10 + 10 + 10 = 30

Very large values use the same rules in the same order — the numbers are simply more complex. Look for such numbers during movie credits where they're often used for copyrights or film release dates.

<u>MCXXIV</u>
M   C   XX   IV
1000 + 100 + 20 + 4 =
1124

<u>MCMXXIV</u>
M   CM   XX   IV
1000 +   900 + 20 + 4 =
1924

<u>MCMXLIX</u>
M   CM   XL   IX
1000 + 900 + 40 + 9 =
1949

<u>MMCMLXXXVIII</u>
MM   CM   LXXX   VIII
2000 + 900 +   80   + 8 =
2988

Practice Set I - 1   Convert to Roman or Arabic numerals as appropriate

1. _____ XX

2. _____ MCLXXIX

3. _____ LXIV

4. _____ XXVI

5. _____ XCIX

6. _____ XXIII

7. _____ CDXLVIII

8. _____ xix

9. _____ MMMCCCXXXIII

10. _____ xxix

11. _____ iv

12. _____ CX

13. _____ III

14. _____ xxiv

15. _____ LVII

16. _____ CDIX

17. _____ xxxii

18. 15 _____

19. 1973 _____

20. 30 _____

21. 9 _____

22. 2435 _____

23. 29 _____

24. 112 _____

25. 49 _____

26. 8 _____

27. 2222 _____

28. 16 _____

29. 4 _____

30. 14 _____

31. 54 _____

32. 11 _____

33. 76 _____

34. 59 _____

Chapter 2
Introduction To Fractions

The actual measurement of many of the quantities with which we deal in the lab, in the home and in business force us to realize that the use of whole numbers alone is not sufficient to represent all information. We are simply compelled to use fractional measurements.

The parts of a fraction are called terms. In any common fraction there are two terms — the Numerator and the Denominator. The *denominator* is the number written below the line of the fraction. It shows into how many equal parts the unit has been divided. In the following fractions, which number is the denominator:

$$a. \frac{2}{3} \quad b. \frac{3}{7} \quad c. \frac{2}{5} \quad d. \frac{1}{16}$$

If your answers are 3, 7, 5, 16, respectively, then you are correct.

Fraction "a" indicates a whole unit has been divided into how many equal parts? ____

If you selected 3, you are correct.

The *Numerator* is the number written above the line of the fraction and shows how many equal parts there are of the unit. In the following fractions, which number is the numerator?

$$a. \frac{1}{16} \quad b. \frac{7}{12} \quad c. \frac{1}{2} \quad d. \frac{3}{8}$$

Your answers should read: 1, 7, 1, 3 respectively

The following figures have been divided into equal parts. A certain number of these parts have been shaded. Write the fraction that indicates what part of each figure is shaded.

(a)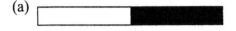

(b)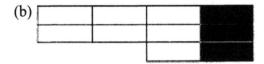

(c)

(d)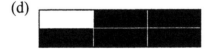

Your answer for "a" should be $1/2$. The denominator 2 indicates the units have been divided into two equal parts. The numerator 1 indicates that only one of the equal parts has been shaded. The correct answer for "b", "c", and "d" is $3/10$, $3/4$ and $5/6$, respectively.

In Practice Set II – 1 express your answers as fractions. Be sure to check your answers and correct errors.

Practice Set II - 1

1. List the shaded parts of each figure in terms of a fraction:

a.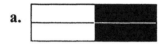

b.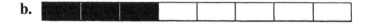

c.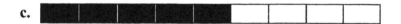

d.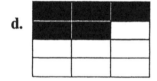

2. There are 12 inches in a foot. Express each of the following as a fraction of a foot:

    a. 1 in. _____   **b.** 5 in. _____   **c.** 11 in. _____   **d.** 7 in. _____

3. There are 36 inches in a yard. Express each of the following as fractions of a yard:

    a. 1 in. _____   **b.** 35 in. _____   **c.** 13 in. _____   **d.** 19 in. _____

4. Express each of the following as fractions of an hour:

    a. 7 min. _____   **b.** 13 min. _____   **c.** 30 min. _____   **d.** 45 min. _____

5. Express each of the problems shown as fractions of a dollar:

    a. 12 cents _____   **b.** 37 cents _____   **c.** 50 cents _____   **d.** 99 cents _____

Common fractions are fractions whose numerators and denominators are whole numbers.

Examples: (i) $\dfrac{1}{2}$ (ii) $\dfrac{16}{9}$ (iii) $\dfrac{2}{3}$ (iv) $\dfrac{5}{4}$

Proper fractions are fractions which are less than one, that is whose numerators are less than the denominators.

Examples: (i) $\dfrac{1}{2}$ (ii) $\dfrac{1}{3}$ (iii) $\dfrac{16}{19}$ (iv) $\dfrac{8}{9}$

Improper fractions have numerators which are equal to or larger than the denominators.

Examples: (i) $\dfrac{11}{6}$ (ii) $\dfrac{24}{23}$ (iii) $\dfrac{4}{3}$ (iv) $\dfrac{8}{5}$

Mixed numbers are numbers composed of a whole number and a fraction.

Examples: (i) $1\dfrac{5}{6}$ (ii) $1\dfrac{1}{23}$ (iii) $1\dfrac{1}{3}$ (iv) $1\dfrac{3}{5}$

Notes:
   (a) Improper fractions can be converted to mixed numbers and vice versa.
   (b) The examples shown for improper fractions correspond in values to those shown for mixed numbers.

Complex fractions are usually "fractions over fractions"; or fractions or mixed numbers in the numerator or the denominator or both.

Examples: i. $\dfrac{1/2}{7/8}$ ii. $\dfrac{3/4}{2/9}$

Reducing fractions, or expressing fractions in lowest terms, is a general practice used everywhere. It makes fractions easier to read and understand.

Example: Which is easiest to understand and use?

$$\frac{1}{3} \quad or \quad \frac{17}{51} \quad or \quad \frac{34}{102}$$ They all have the same value.

In order for a fraction to be reduced to lowest terms, both the numerator and denominator must be divisible by the same number.

$\frac{5}{10}$ ⟵ reduces to 1 when the numerator is divided by 5

        ⟵ reduces to 2 when the denominator is divided by 5

$\frac{3}{12}$ ⟵ divided by 3 = 1

        ⟵ divided by 3 = 4

Note that the value of the fraction does not change.

$$\frac{5}{10} = \frac{1}{2} \qquad\qquad\qquad \frac{3}{12} = \frac{1}{4}$$

For the smaller fractions, the number used to divide is generally easy to determine.

Examples:

(i) $\dfrac{4}{8} \quad \dfrac{\text{divide by 4}}{\text{divide by 4}} \quad = \dfrac{1}{2}$ (ii) $\dfrac{3}{9} \quad \dfrac{\text{divide by 3}}{\text{divide by 3}} \quad = \dfrac{1}{3}$

However, when the number is larger, it can be more difficult to determine a single number that reduces both the numerator and denominator. Successive applications of the procedure can be used instead. The method remains the same and can be performed in multiple steps. First, find a number which will divide into both numerator and denominator. Then, inspect the resulting fraction to see if it can be further reduced.

Example: $\dfrac{16}{64}\left(\dfrac{\div 4}{\div 4}\right) = \dfrac{4}{16}\left(\dfrac{\div 4}{\div 4}\right) = \dfrac{1}{4}$

This example was performed in two steps. It could have been completed in one step if it had been observed that both numerator and denominator were divisible by 16.

$$\dfrac{16}{64}\left(\dfrac{\div 16}{\div 16}\right) = \dfrac{1}{4}$$

Some helpful hints are:
    (a) If both numbers are even, then they will be divisible by 2.
    (b) If the sum of the digits is divisible by 3, the number is divisible by 3.
    (c) If both numbers end in 0 or 5, then they are divisible by 5.

This is often a trial-and-error procedure until proficiency is acquired. A good knowledge of both multiplication and division tables is extremely helpful.

Practice Set II-2   Reduce each of the following fractions to the lowest terms:

1. $\dfrac{3}{5} =$ 2. $\dfrac{2}{4} =$ 3. $\dfrac{4}{8} =$ 4. $\dfrac{12}{16} =$

5. $\dfrac{12}{3} =$ 6. $\dfrac{9}{27} =$ 7. $\dfrac{13}{26} =$ 8. $\dfrac{21}{24} =$

9. $\dfrac{8}{9} =$ 10. $\dfrac{20}{30} =$ 11. $\dfrac{45}{81} =$ 12. $\dfrac{22}{77} =$

Improper Fractions and Mixed Numbers

To change improper fractions to mixed numbers, divide the denominator into the numerator for a whole number value. After dividing, the remainder becomes the numerator of the fraction. The denominator of the fraction part is the same as the denominator of the imroper fraction.

Examples:

(i) $\dfrac{7}{5}$ divide 5 into 7 which equals 1 with remainder of 2. This 2 becomes the numerator and the denominator stays at 5 $= 1\dfrac{2}{5}$

(ii)   Convert $\dfrac{12}{5}$ to a mixed number.

$\dfrac{12}{5}$ divide 5 into 12 $\begin{array}{r} 2 \\ 5\overline{)12} \\ -10 \\ \hline 2 \end{array}$ write the mixed number

determine the remainder (2) $= 2\dfrac{2}{5}$

(iii) $\dfrac{6}{5} \longrightarrow$ $\begin{array}{r} 1 \\ 5\overline{)6} \\ 5 \\ \hline 1 \end{array}$ = remainder $= 1\dfrac{1}{5}$

(iv) $\dfrac{19}{6} \longrightarrow$ $\begin{array}{r} 3 \\ 6\overline{)19} \\ 18 \\ \hline 1 \end{array}$ = remainder $\longrightarrow$ $= 3\dfrac{1}{6}$

(v) $\dfrac{18}{4} \longrightarrow$ $\begin{array}{r} 4 \\ 4\overline{)18} \\ 16 \\ \hline 2 \end{array}$ $\longrightarrow = 4\dfrac{2}{4} \longrightarrow = 4\dfrac{1}{2}$

divide   rewrite   reduce to lowest terms

To change mixed numbers to improper fractions, the whole number portion is multiplied by the denominator of the fraction. This product is added to the original numerator and the sum becomes the new numerator.

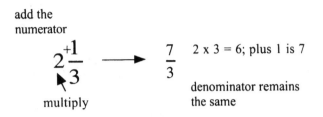

add the
numerator

$$2\overset{+1}{\underset{3}{}} \longrightarrow \frac{7}{3}$$ 2 x 3 = 6; plus 1 is 7

multiply   denominator remains
                                        the same

Example: $3\frac{4}{5} = \frac{19}{5}$ 5 x 3 = 15; plus 4 is 19

                              denominator
                              remains the same

Practice Set II - 3

Convert to a mixed number or an improper fraction as appropriate.

1. $\dfrac{10}{3} =$

2. $\dfrac{17}{5} =$

3. $\dfrac{25}{4} =$

4. $\dfrac{33}{8} =$

5. $\dfrac{35}{16} =$

6. $\dfrac{12}{3} =$

7. $4\dfrac{1}{3} =$

8. $16\dfrac{1}{2} =$

9. $1\dfrac{9}{10} =$

10. $5\dfrac{2}{7} =$

11. $3\dfrac{8}{9} =$

12. $12\dfrac{3}{4} =$

Practice Set II - 4

1. Reduce each fraction to lowest terms:

a. $\dfrac{11}{44}$ **b.** $\dfrac{17}{102}$ **c.** $\dfrac{24}{25}$

d. $\dfrac{12}{48}$ **e.** $\dfrac{48}{96}$ **f.** $\dfrac{5}{30}$

g. $\dfrac{4}{32}$ **h.** $\dfrac{3}{27}$

2. Change to improper fractions:

a. $8\dfrac{7}{8}$ **b.** $2\dfrac{13}{18}$ **c.** $7\dfrac{5}{6}$

d. $3\dfrac{5}{8}$ **e.** $4\dfrac{11}{12}$ **f.** $7\dfrac{5}{7}$

g. $6\dfrac{8}{9}$ **h.** $2\dfrac{5}{8}$

3. Change to mixed numbers:

a. $\dfrac{51}{17}$ b. $\dfrac{48}{7}$ c. $\dfrac{55}{9}$

d. $\dfrac{64}{9}$ e. $\dfrac{85}{4}$ f. $\dfrac{25}{7}$

g. $\dfrac{21}{5}$ h. $\dfrac{21}{4}$

Chapter 3
Multiplication and Division of Fractions

Multiplication of Fractions

Multiplication can be defined as successive addition. That is, 3 x $^1/_8$ means $\frac{1}{8} + \frac{1}{8} + \frac{1}{8}$ or $^3/_8$.

Example:

6 x $^2/_3$ means $\quad \frac{2}{3} + \frac{2}{3} + \frac{2}{3} + \frac{2}{3} + \frac{2}{3} + \frac{2}{3} \quad$ or $\quad \frac{2}{3} + \frac{2}{3} + \frac{2}{3} + \frac{2}{3} + \frac{2}{3} + \frac{2}{3} = \frac{12}{3} = 4$

$$\underbrace{\qquad\qquad\qquad\qquad}_{6 \text{ times}}$$

Multiplication is a short cut for repeated addition and can be a time saver in the clinic. Notice in the examples given, we have been multiplying a whole number times a fraction. Fractions are multiplied across numerators and denominators. Since any whole number can be written with the numeral one (1) as a denominator, examine the following examples of multiplying fractions.

Examples: $\quad 4 \times \frac{2}{5} \quad$ is the same as $\quad \frac{4}{1} \times \frac{2}{5} \quad$ and $\quad \frac{2}{3} \times 5 = \frac{2}{3} \times \frac{5}{1}$

Example Multiplying:

$$\longrightarrow \frac{4}{1} \times \frac{2}{5} = \frac{4 \times 2}{1 \times 5} = \frac{8}{5} = 1\frac{3}{5} \quad \textit{always reduce to lowest terms}$$

$$\frac{2}{3} \times 5 = \frac{2}{3} \times \frac{5}{1} = \frac{2 \times 5}{3 \times 1} = \frac{10}{3} = 3\frac{1}{3} \quad \text{which is the same as} \quad \frac{2}{3} + \frac{2}{3} + \frac{2}{3} + \frac{2}{3} + \frac{2}{3} = \frac{10}{3} = 3\frac{1}{3}$$

Practice Set III – 1

Multiply the following fractions and whole numbers:

1. $4 \times \frac{1}{3} =$ 2. $5 \times \frac{1}{4} =$ 3. $7 \times \frac{1}{2} =$ 4. $18 \times \frac{2}{9} =$

5. $4 \times \frac{5}{7} =$ 6. $5 \times \frac{1}{2} =$ 7. $\frac{1}{3} \times 5 =$ 8. $\frac{5}{6} \times 10 =$

Multiplying fractions by fractions is done in the same manner. Multiply numerator by numerator and denominator by denominator. Simplify.

Examples:

(i) $\frac{1}{3} \times \frac{1}{2} = \frac{1 \times 1}{3 \times 2} = \frac{1}{6}$ (ii) $\frac{4}{9} \times \frac{2}{5} = \frac{4 \times 2}{9 \times 5} = \frac{8}{45}$

Practice Set III – 2

Multiply the following fractions. Be sure to reduce where necessary.

1. $\dfrac{1}{3} \times \dfrac{1}{3} =$

2. $\dfrac{1}{4} \times \dfrac{1}{4} =$

3. $\dfrac{1}{3} \times \dfrac{1}{4} =$

4. $\dfrac{2}{9} \times \dfrac{2}{3} =$

5. $\dfrac{3}{4} \times \dfrac{2}{5} =$

6. $\dfrac{2}{5} \times \dfrac{3}{5} =$

7. $\dfrac{3}{4} \times \dfrac{5}{8} =$

8. $\dfrac{7}{8} \times \dfrac{3}{5} =$

Now, we're going to examine a short cut that can frequently be used when multiplying fractions. Sometimes we can divide a numerator and a denominator each by the same factor and thus simplify the multiplication. This process is referred to as cancellation, since we "cancel" one or more of the factors being multiplied. This simplifies the whole process. Unfortunately, the term cancellation can confuse students; furthermore, it is not a very good description of the math concepts that allow one to "cancel".

Cancellation gets its name from the mechanics of the process as well as the effect. But, we're not really "canceling" anything – or somehow performing math magic. Rather it is based upon the principle that any number divided by itself is 1. Also, a number multiplied by 1 remains the same number. Thus,

$$\frac{5}{6} \times \frac{6}{7} = \frac{5 \boxed{\times 6}}{7 \boxed{\times 6}}^{\,= 1} = \frac{5}{7} \times 1 = \frac{5}{7}$$

As you can see, the sixes "cancel" each other; hence the term cancellation. The result is a way to "short-cut" multiplication of fractions.

$$\frac{5}{\cancel{6}} \times \frac{\cancel{6}}{7} = \frac{5}{7}$$

When can this technique be applied? Think of a bow tie. If the terms you wish to cancel are at any of the points (the darkened circles) on the bow tie, then cancellation will "work" as long as those points are connected by a line (as shown.)

Here are some additional *examples:*

(i) $\dfrac{2}{\cancel{3}_1} \times \dfrac{\cancel{3}^1}{5} = \dfrac{2}{5}$

Threes connected

(ii) $\dfrac{3}{\cancel{4}_1} \times \dfrac{\cancel{8}^2}{11} = \dfrac{6}{11}$ since 4 goes into 4 one time and 4 goes into 8 two times

Four and eight lie at points connected by a line

(iii) $\dfrac{\cancel{5}^1}{\cancel{7}_1} \times \dfrac{\cancel{14}^2}{\cancel{25}_5} = \dfrac{2}{5}$

seven into 14 twice and 5 into 25 five times

(iv) $\dfrac{2}{3} \times \dfrac{2}{5} = \dfrac{4}{15}$ Remember the bow tie? The 2's won't cancel!

(v) $\dfrac{^2\cancel{4}}{7}\times\dfrac{3}{\cancel{6}_3}=\dfrac{6}{21}=\dfrac{2}{7}$ 2 divides into 4 two times
and into 6 three times

$\dfrac{^2\cancel{4}}{7}\times\dfrac{\cancel{3}^1}{\cancel{6}_{\cancel{3}_1}}=\dfrac{2}{7}$ Same as above, but shown
with the threes canceling
each other; multiple
cancellations are okay

(vi) $2\times\dfrac{3}{8}\times\dfrac{6}{11}$

$\dfrac{^1\cancel{2}}{1}\times\dfrac{3}{\cancel{8}_{\cancel{2}_{\cancel{4}}}}\times\dfrac{\cancel{6}^3}{11}$ Multiple cancellations are allowed.
Here, two divides evenly into itself
and 8. It divides again into 4 and 6.

Multiply across numerators
and denominators for the result.

$\dfrac{1}{1}\times\dfrac{3}{2}\times\dfrac{3}{11}=\dfrac{9}{22}$

Practice Set III – 3

Multiply each of the following. Use the "cancellation" technique wherever possible.

1. $\dfrac{4}{9}\times\dfrac{3}{5}=$ 2. $\dfrac{2}{5}\times\dfrac{3}{10}=$ 3. $\dfrac{2}{5}\times\dfrac{3}{8}=$ 4. $\dfrac{4}{5}\times\dfrac{3}{10}=$

5. $\dfrac{3}{4}\times\dfrac{4}{5}=$ 6. $\dfrac{9}{10}\times\dfrac{4}{27}=$ 7. $\dfrac{2}{5}\times\dfrac{5}{8}=$ 8. $\dfrac{5}{12}\times\dfrac{4}{15}=$

9. $\dfrac{3}{8}\times\dfrac{4}{9}=$ 10. $\dfrac{7}{8}\times\dfrac{2}{7}=$ 11. $\dfrac{2}{3}\times\dfrac{3}{4}\times\dfrac{12}{15}=$ 12. $\dfrac{6}{7}\times\dfrac{14}{15}\times\dfrac{5}{8}=$

In the preceding sections, you have learned how to multiply fractions by whole numbers and whole numbers by fractions, how to multiply fractions by fractions and the technique of cancellation. Now, we'll learn how to multiply mixed numbers.

The only way to multiply mixed numbers is to first convert each mixed number to an improper fraction.

To multiply a mixed number by a whole number, change the mixed number to an improper fraction and multiply; cancel if possible; and reduce to lowest terms if possible.

Examples:

(i) $4\dfrac{2}{3} \times 9 = \dfrac{14}{3} \times 9 = \dfrac{14}{\underset{1}{\cancel{3}}} \times \dfrac{\overset{3}{\cancel{9}}}{1} = \dfrac{42}{1} = 42$ (ii) $3\dfrac{1}{2} \times 8 = \dfrac{7}{\underset{1}{\cancel{2}}} \times \dfrac{\overset{4}{\cancel{8}}}{1} = 28$

Practice Set III – 4
Multiply.

1. $5\dfrac{1}{3} \times 6 =$ 2. $1\dfrac{1}{4} \times 4 =$ 3. $8 \times 2\dfrac{3}{4} =$

4. $2 \times 5\dfrac{3}{4} =$ 5. $6 \times 2\dfrac{1}{5} =$ 6. $1\dfrac{2}{5} \times 3 =$

When both terms are mixed numbers change both mixed numbers to improper fractions and multiply.

Example: $4\dfrac{1}{8} \times 2\dfrac{2}{11} = \dfrac{\cancel{33}^{3}}{\cancel{8}_{1}} \times \dfrac{\cancel{24}^{3}}{\cancel{11}_{1}} = \dfrac{9}{1} = 9$

7. $2\dfrac{2}{3} \times 3\dfrac{1}{2} =$ 8. $3\dfrac{1}{3} \times 3\dfrac{2}{7} =$ 9. $4\dfrac{1}{5} \times 2\dfrac{1}{3} =$ 10. $7\dfrac{2}{3} \times 1\dfrac{1}{2} =$

11. $8\dfrac{1}{3} \times 6\dfrac{3}{4} =$ 12. $5\dfrac{1}{6} \times 2\dfrac{1}{2} =$ 13. $2\dfrac{3}{8} \times 3\dfrac{8}{16} =$ 14. $4\dfrac{1}{3} \times 3\dfrac{1}{4} =$

Applications: most of the problems you encounter in the working world are "word problems". That is, someone communicates information, verbally or written, and that information is used to solve some problem.

Practice Set III – 5

Solve the following application problems.

1. What is the total weight of 5 boxes each weighing 8 $^1/_4$ pounds?

2. Calculate the total weight of 12 steel cages if each cage is 11 feet long and each cage weighs 2 $^1/_8$ lb. per foot.

3. What is the weight of 12 operating instruments, if each one weighs 1 $^3/_4$ pounds?

4. A gallon of a certain solution requires 5 $^7/_8$ ounces of a particular chemical. How many ounces of that chemical are needed to make three gallons of solution?

Division of Fractions

Draw a line 6 inches long like the one you see here.

_____

If you cut this line into $^1/_4$ inch pieces, how many would you get? Mark it off and count them. You should have 24 vertical marks. Another way to find out the number of vertical marks needed is to divide 6 by $^1/_4$.

Example:

$$6 \div \frac{1}{4} \ =$$

The number or fraction to the right is called the divisor. In this example $^1/_4$ is the divisor.

$$6 \times \frac{4}{1} \ =$$

To divide by a fraction invert the divisor and multiply. (The answer is 24.)

When the numerator and denominator change places, we say the fraction has been *Inverted.* To invert means to turn over. A whole number like 5 when inverted becomes $^1/_5$ therefore $^1/_5$ is the *reciprocal* of 5. When dividing fractions, what we really do is multiply by the reciprocal.

Example: The reciprocal of $\dfrac{1}{5}$ is 5.   The reciprocal of $\dfrac{2}{3}$ is $\dfrac{3}{2}$

$$3 \div \frac{1}{5} = \frac{3}{1} \times \frac{5}{1} = \frac{15}{1} = 15 \qquad 8 \div \frac{2}{3} = \frac{8}{1} \times \frac{3}{2} = \frac{24}{2} = 12$$

To divide fractions invert the divisor and multiply. If possible, reduce the result.

Examples: (i) $\dfrac{5}{6} \div \dfrac{5}{7}$

Divide fractions by inverting the divisor and multiplying. You may use cancellation techniques. Simplify if possible.

$$\dfrac{{}^1\cancel{5}}{6} \times \dfrac{7}{\cancel{5}_{1}} = \dfrac{7}{6} = 1\dfrac{1}{6}$$

(ii) $\dfrac{2}{3} \div \dfrac{1}{2}$

$$\dfrac{2}{3} \times \dfrac{2}{1} = \dfrac{4}{3} = 1\dfrac{1}{3}$$

(iii) $\dfrac{7}{12} \div \dfrac{3}{4}$ *or*

$$\dfrac{7}{\cancel{12}_{3}} \times \dfrac{\cancel{4}^{1}}{3} = \dfrac{7}{9}$$

$\dfrac{7}{12} \div \dfrac{3}{4}$

$$\dfrac{7}{12} \times \dfrac{4}{3} = \dfrac{28}{36} = \dfrac{7}{9}$$

Practice Set III – 6

Divide the following fractions.

1. $\dfrac{2}{3} \div \dfrac{4}{5} =$ 2. $\dfrac{5}{16} \div \dfrac{5}{32} =$ 3. $\dfrac{4}{5} \div \dfrac{2}{3} =$ 4. $\dfrac{2}{9} \div \dfrac{3}{4} =$

5. $\dfrac{5}{12} \div \dfrac{3}{4} =$ 6. $\dfrac{9}{16} \div \dfrac{3}{8} =$ 7. $\dfrac{7}{8} \div \dfrac{5}{12} =$ 8. $\dfrac{3}{16} \div \dfrac{9}{32} =$

Application:

9. A cafe owner used a $3/4$ pound can of pepper to fill the pepper shakers. Each shaker can hold $1/64$ pound of pepper. In this way, how many shakers would she fill from the $3/4$ pound can?

Dividing a whole number by a fraction uses the same technique. Invert the divisor and multiply. It may be helpful to write the whole number as a fraction when you do this.

Examples: (i) $8 \div \dfrac{2}{5}$ Write the whole number using 1 as a denominator. Invert the divisor and multiply. You may use cancellation if you desire.

$$\frac{8}{1} \div \frac{2}{5}$$

$$\frac{8}{1} \times \frac{5}{2} = \frac{40}{2} = 20$$

(ii) $10 \div \dfrac{5}{7}$

$$\frac{10}{1} \div \frac{5}{7}$$

$$\frac{{}^{2}\cancel{10}}{1} \times \frac{7}{\cancel{5}_{1}} = \frac{14}{1} = 14$$

Practice Set III – 7

Solve.

1. $5 \div \dfrac{1}{3} =$ **2.** $4 \div \dfrac{1}{4} =$ **3.** $8 \div \dfrac{1}{2} =$

4. $25 \div \dfrac{5}{7} =$ **5.** $18 \div \dfrac{4}{3} =$ **6.** $45 \div \dfrac{10}{9} =$

7. $40 \div \dfrac{3}{8} =$ **8.** $96 \div \dfrac{23}{24} =$ **9.** $63 \div \dfrac{3}{10} =$

When dividing fractions by whole numbers, follow the same procedure. Make the divisor a fraction, then invert it and multiply.

Example:

$$\frac{8}{9} \div 2 =$$

$$\frac{8}{9} \div \frac{2}{1} =$$ Notice the use the reciprocal and multiplication.

$$\frac{8}{9} \times \frac{1}{2} =$$

$$\frac{8}{18} = \frac{4}{9}$$ Always reduce to lowest terms.

Practice Set III – 8
   Divide.

1. $\dfrac{7}{8} \div 5 =$

2. $\dfrac{2}{3} \div 6 =$

3. $\dfrac{7}{16} \div 7 =$

4. $\dfrac{5}{8} \div 2 =$

5. $\dfrac{9}{11} \div 3 =$

6. $\dfrac{1}{4} \div 4 =$

When multiplying mixed numbers we first had to change any mixed numbers to improper fractions. The same procedure must be followed when dividing mixed numbers. To divide fractions involving mixed numbers change the mixed number to an improper fraction; invert the divisor, multiply, cancel where possible, reduce as necessary.

Examples:

(i) $3\dfrac{1}{2} \div 4$

             change the mixed number to
             an improper fraction

    $\dfrac{7}{2} \div 4$

             change to multiplication and use
             the reciprocal of the divisor

    $\dfrac{7}{2} \times \dfrac{1}{4} = \dfrac{7}{8}$

(ii) $5\dfrac{1}{3} \div 2\dfrac{2}{3}$

             change mixed numbers to
             improper fractions

    $\dfrac{16}{3} \div \dfrac{8}{3}$

             invert the divisor
             and multiply

    $\dfrac{16}{3} \times \dfrac{3}{8}$

             multiply and simplify

$$\dfrac{\overset{2}{\cancel{16}}}{\underset{1}{\cancel{3}}} \times \dfrac{\overset{1}{\cancel{3}}}{\underset{1}{\cancel{8}}} = \dfrac{2}{1} = 2$$

Note the use of cancellation techniques.

Practice Set III – 9
   Divide.

1. $6\dfrac{2}{3} \div \dfrac{1}{4} =$
        2. $5\dfrac{3}{5} \div 7 =$
        3. $4\dfrac{1}{3} \div 10 =$
        4. $\dfrac{3}{5} \div \dfrac{9}{10} =$

5. $\dfrac{5}{8} \div 2\dfrac{1}{2} =$

6. $4\dfrac{1}{5} \div 1\dfrac{3}{4} =$

7. $30 \div 1\dfrac{2}{3} =$

8. $17\dfrac{1}{2} \div 3\dfrac{1}{2} =$

9. $6\dfrac{2}{5} \div 5\dfrac{1}{3} =$

10. $85 \div 4\dfrac{1}{4} =$

Practice Set III – 10

Review. Perform the indicated operation and simplify.

1. $\dfrac{7}{8} \times \dfrac{8}{9} =$

2. $1\dfrac{2}{3} \times \dfrac{3}{10} =$

3. $\dfrac{4}{5} \times \dfrac{1}{2} =$

4. $2 \times \dfrac{5}{8} \times 1\dfrac{3}{4} =$

5. $\dfrac{6}{8} \times \dfrac{2}{3} =$

6. $3\dfrac{1}{2} \times \dfrac{12}{8} \times 1\dfrac{1}{2} =$

7. $\dfrac{17}{51} \times \dfrac{1}{2} =$

8. $\dfrac{3}{3} \times \dfrac{2}{2} \times \dfrac{5}{5} =$

9. $\dfrac{9}{10} \times \dfrac{5}{3} =$

10. $\dfrac{1}{2} \div \dfrac{1}{4} =$

11. $\dfrac{9}{10} \times 1\dfrac{2}{3} =$

12. $\dfrac{1}{6} \div \dfrac{1}{8} =$

13. $1\dfrac{2}{3} \times 3\dfrac{1}{5} =$

14. $\dfrac{1}{3} \div \dfrac{2}{7} =$

15. $24 \times \dfrac{1}{2} =$

16. $1\dfrac{2}{5} \div \dfrac{3}{10} =$

17. $24 \times \dfrac{1}{3} =$

18. $2\dfrac{6}{10} \div \dfrac{10}{14} =$

19. $24 \times \dfrac{2}{3} =$

20. $8\dfrac{8}{10} \div \dfrac{11}{5} =$

21. $24 \times \dfrac{3}{3} =$

22. $2\dfrac{3}{4} \div \dfrac{11}{16} =$

23. $\dfrac{3}{4} \times \dfrac{2}{3} \times \dfrac{1}{2} =$

24. $3\dfrac{4}{5} \div 6\dfrac{7}{8} =$

25. $1\dfrac{2}{3} \div 4\dfrac{5}{6} =$

26. $9 \div \dfrac{1}{3} =$

27. $4 \div \dfrac{1}{2} =$

28. $\dfrac{1}{2} \div \dfrac{1}{4} =$

29. $\dfrac{2}{5} \div 1\dfrac{1}{4} =$

30. $\dfrac{8}{11} \div \dfrac{16}{22} =$

31. $4\dfrac{3}{5} \div \dfrac{23}{30} =$

32. $\dfrac{3}{3} \div \dfrac{2}{2} =$

33. $2\dfrac{1}{2} \div 2\dfrac{1}{2} =$

Chapter 4
Addition and Subtraction of Fractions

Addition of Fractions

Adding fractions with common denominators

To add or subtract fractions, a common denominator is required. To add fractions with a common denominator, add the numerators and write this sum over the common denominator.

Example:

add the numerators

$$\frac{1}{5} + \frac{2}{5} = \frac{1+2}{5} = \frac{3}{5}$$

retain the common denominator

The numerators 1 and 2 are added and their sum, 3, is written over the common denominator, 5. Reduce any fraction to lowest terms, if possible; and convert any improper fraction to a mixed number.

Practice Set IV – 1

Add the following fractions. Be sure to reduce where necessary:

1. $\dfrac{3}{8} + \dfrac{4}{8} =$

   2. $\dfrac{9}{16} + \dfrac{1}{16} =$

   3. $\dfrac{3}{5} + \dfrac{1}{5} =$

   4. $\begin{array}{r} \dfrac{7}{16} \\ +\dfrac{5}{16} \\ \hline \end{array}$

5. $\begin{array}{r} \dfrac{1}{7} \\ +\dfrac{2}{7} \\ \hline \end{array}$

   6. $\begin{array}{r} \dfrac{5}{8} \\ \dfrac{1}{8} \\ +\dfrac{3}{8} \\ \hline \end{array}$

   7. $\begin{array}{r} \dfrac{2}{16} \\ \dfrac{11}{16} \\ +\dfrac{7}{16} \\ \hline \end{array}$

Adding Fractions with Different Denominators

Fractions cannot be added unless they have a common denominator. Fractions have a common denominator when all their denominators are the same, as $\dfrac{5}{8}, \dfrac{7}{8}$, and $\dfrac{3}{8}$.

Example:

$$\dfrac{2}{3} + \dfrac{3}{4} + \dfrac{1}{2} = ?$$ Fractions without common denominators.

When the denominators are not the same, make them the same. First determine a common denominator, preferably, the **LCD** (*least common denominator*). That is, find the smallest number into which all the given denominators will divide evenly. In this example, the lowest number into which all the denominators (3, 4, and 2) will evenly divide is 12. This will be the least common denominator.

The next step is to adjust the denominator in each fraction to a common denominator.

$$\frac{2}{3} \times \frac{}{4} = \frac{}{12}$$

$$\frac{3}{4} \times \frac{}{3} = \frac{}{12}$$

$$\frac{1}{2} \times \frac{}{6} = \frac{}{12}$$

by multiplying each denominator by a different number, we achieve the common denominator in each case

Then adjust the numerators in a similar fashion. Recall that any number multiplied by 1 is the same number – its value doesn't change. Furthermore, any fraction which has the same numerator and denominator is equal to 1. Since each denominator was multiplied by a different number in order to reach 12, multiply the numerators by that same number in each case.

$$\frac{2}{3} \times \frac{4}{4} = \frac{8}{12}$$

$$\frac{3}{4} \times \frac{3}{3} = \frac{9}{12}$$

$$\frac{1}{2} \times \frac{6}{6} = \frac{6}{12}$$

multiplying each fraction by the same number with which we achieved the denominator, adjusts the numerator.

We now have a common denominator and the fractions can be added.

$$\frac{2}{3} \times \frac{4}{4} = \frac{8}{12}$$

$$\frac{3}{4} \times \frac{3}{3} = \frac{9}{12}$$

$$+ \quad \frac{1}{2} \times \frac{6}{6} = \frac{6}{12}$$

$$\frac{23}{12}$$

Reduce to simplest form $\frac{23}{12} = 1\frac{11}{12}$

Another look at the same problem: $\frac{8}{12} + \frac{9}{12} + \frac{6}{12} = \frac{8+9+6}{12} = \frac{23}{12} = 1\frac{11}{12}$

Practice Set IV – 2

Add the fractions. Remember to find the LCD; reduce to simplest form where possible.

1. $\frac{1}{12} + \frac{1}{4} =$ 2. $\frac{1}{6} + \frac{1}{3} =$ 3. $\frac{1}{2} + \frac{1}{6} =$

4. $\begin{array}{r} \frac{1}{4} \\ + \frac{1}{2} \\ \hline \end{array}$ 5. $\begin{array}{r} \frac{5}{12} \\ + \frac{1}{4} \\ \hline \end{array}$ 6. $\begin{array}{r} \frac{3}{8} \\ + \frac{1}{4} \\ \hline \end{array}$

7. $\dfrac{1}{8}$

$+\dfrac{1}{2}$

___

8. $\dfrac{3}{6}$

$+\dfrac{1}{3}$

___

9. $\dfrac{1}{8}$

$+\dfrac{1}{4}$

___

10. $\dfrac{1}{3}$

$+\dfrac{1}{2}$

___

11. $\dfrac{1}{7}+\dfrac{1}{2}=$

12. $\dfrac{3}{8}+\dfrac{3}{4}=$

13. $\dfrac{1}{16}$

$\dfrac{1}{24}$

$\dfrac{3}{48}$

$+\dfrac{1}{6}$

___

14. $\dfrac{1}{4}$

$\dfrac{3}{8}$

$\dfrac{3}{4}$

$+\dfrac{5}{6}$

___

15. $\dfrac{5}{6}$

$\dfrac{1}{8}$

$+\dfrac{2}{3}$

___

Here is a technique for finding the least common denominator. Suppose the problems has denominators of 6, 8 and 10. Using division without remainder, that is, divide evenly:

LCD = 120

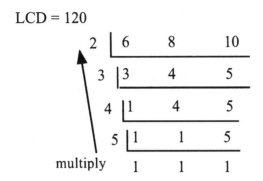

Divide by any number that will divide evenly into any of the denominators. If it will not divide evenly, don't divide at all. The goal is to get all "1"s along the bottom row. You can see that first our denominators were divided by 2, followed by 3. This left a 1, 4 and 5.

Continue to divide using values that divide with no remainders. Once all 1s have been achieved along the bottom row, multiply up the "ladder" to find the LCD. In this case, it's 5 x 4 x 3 x 2 = 120.

Example: Denominators are 6, 14 and 5.

LCD = 210

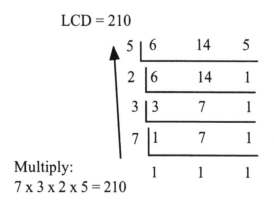

Divide. Continue the process until the last row contains only 1s. Then multiply the numbers along the left side.

Adding Mixed Numbers

A mixed number is a number composed of a whole number and a fraction taken together, such as $3\frac{2}{5}$ or $1\frac{2}{3}$. To add mixed numbers — add the whole numbers and the fractions separately and combine the results. (*It is not necessary to convert to improper fractions as when multiplying or dividing.*) Simplify and reduce as needed.

Example:

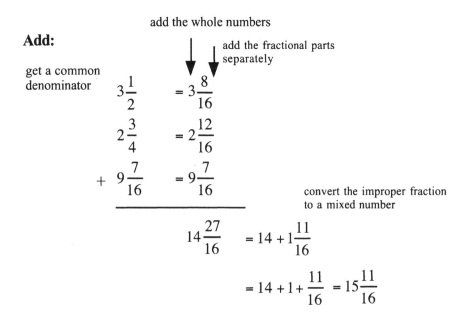

In this example, the fractions were changed to 16ths (for a common denominator) and added for a sum of $\frac{27}{16}$, which simplifies to $1\frac{11}{16}$. The sum of the whole numbers was 14. Combining these results yields the solution $15\frac{11}{16}$.

Another procedure for adding mixed numbers involves changing all the mixed numbers to improper fractions before adding. That procedure, while correct, tends to involve more steps thus increasing the possibility for error. If you know how to do this procedure, and are comfortable with doing it, then you are welcome to do so. In math, there are often several ways to a solution. Rarely, though, is there only one "right" way. Any method that is mathematically sound and achieves the desired result is acceptable.

Practice Set IV – 3
  Add.

1. $5\dfrac{1}{3}$

   $+\ 8\dfrac{1}{12}$
   _____

2. $4\dfrac{3}{5}$

   $+\ 6\dfrac{1}{10}$
   _____

3. $7\dfrac{1}{2}$

   $+\ 12\dfrac{1}{8}$
   _____

4. $8\dfrac{3}{10}$

   $+\ 9\dfrac{2}{5}$
   _____

5. $8\dfrac{1}{2}$

   $+\ 7\dfrac{1}{4}$
   _____

6. $14\dfrac{1}{6}$

   $+\ 6\dfrac{1}{3}$
   _____

7. $15\dfrac{1}{10}$

   $+\ 7\dfrac{1}{2}$
   _____

8. $9\dfrac{3}{8}$

   $+\ 8\dfrac{1}{4}$
   _____

9. $6\dfrac{6}{16}$

   $+\ 7\dfrac{1}{8}$
   _____

10. $12\frac{1}{4}$

     $+7\frac{1}{12}$
     _____

11. $6\frac{7}{10}$

     $+8\frac{4}{5}$
     _____

12. $4\frac{3}{5}$

     $+7\frac{11}{15}$
     _____

13. $9\frac{5}{6}$

     $+6\frac{2}{3}$
     _____

14. $7\frac{1}{2}$

     $+9\frac{3}{8}$
     _____

15. $3\frac{1}{9}$

     $+5\frac{2}{3}$
     _____

Adding Improper Fractions

Improper fractions can be added in two ways: (1) Convert the improper fraction(s) to mixed numbers and add as previously shown; or (2) Determine the common denominator, add the fractions and then convert the answer to a mixed number.

Example:

$$\frac{3}{2} = \frac{9}{6}$$ Determine LCD, adjust numerators and add

$$\frac{5}{3} = \frac{10}{6}$$

$$+\frac{7}{6} = \frac{7}{6}$$
_____

$$\frac{26}{6} = 4\frac{2}{6} = 4\frac{1}{3}$$

Convert to mixed number and reduce to lowest terms

Practice Set IV – 4

Add the following.

1. $\dfrac{17}{16}$
    $\dfrac{9}{8}$
    $+\dfrac{3}{2}$

2. $\dfrac{3}{2}$
    $\dfrac{5}{4}$
    $+\dfrac{11}{8}$

3. $\dfrac{7}{5}$
    $\dfrac{9}{4}$
    $+\dfrac{12}{10}$

4. $\dfrac{27}{9}$
    $\dfrac{24}{8}$
    $+\dfrac{3}{2}$

Combinations of mixed numbers, whole numbers, and fractions of numbers — common and improper — are combined similarly.

Example: Sum. $\dfrac{2}{3} + 7 + 4\dfrac{1}{5} + \dfrac{7}{2} =$

$\dfrac{2}{3} = \dfrac{20}{30}$

$+\,7 \;=\; 7$ Determine common denominator.
                         Sum and simplify.
$+\,4\dfrac{1}{5} = 4\dfrac{6}{30}$

$+\,\dfrac{7}{2} = \dfrac{105}{30}$

$\qquad\qquad 11\dfrac{131}{30} = 11 + 4\dfrac{11}{30} = 15\dfrac{11}{30}$

Practice Set IV – 5

Add the following.

1. $1\dfrac{3}{4}$
   $\dfrac{5}{3}$
   $+\dfrac{1}{2}$
   _____

2. $4\dfrac{3}{5}$
   $6\dfrac{3}{8}$
   $+\dfrac{23}{20}$
   _____

3. $2\dfrac{1}{2}$
   $3\dfrac{1}{2}$
   $+2\dfrac{2}{3}$
   _____

4. $4\dfrac{3}{16}$
   $3\dfrac{2}{5}$
   $2\dfrac{1}{4}$
   $+1\dfrac{1}{2}$
   _____

Subtraction of Fractions

Subtracting fractions is very similar to adding fractions except now the arithmetic operation is subtraction. Nearly everything else you've learned about adding fractions applies to subtracting them as well.

To subtract proper fractions with like denominators, subtract the numerators and place the result over the common denominator. Remember to reduce or simplify if possible.

Example:

Vertically

$$\frac{9}{16}$$
$$-\frac{7}{16}$$
$$\overline{}$$
$$\frac{2}{16}=\frac{1}{8}$$

Or Horizontally

$$\frac{9}{16}-\frac{7}{16}=\frac{9-7}{16}=\frac{2}{16}=\frac{1}{8}$$

Practice Set IV – 6

Subtract the following fractions with like denominators.

1. $\dfrac{2}{3}$
    $-\dfrac{1}{3}$

2. $\dfrac{5}{6}$
    $-\dfrac{4}{6}$

3. $\dfrac{8}{11}$
    $-\dfrac{1}{11}$

4. $\dfrac{13}{16}$
    $-\dfrac{5}{16}$

When subtracting fractions with unlike denominators, first determine a common denominator, then adjust the numerators as needed and subtract. This is exactly as you have done when adding fractions.

Examples:

$$\dfrac{5}{8} = \dfrac{5}{8}$$
$$-\dfrac{1}{4} = -\dfrac{2}{8}$$
$$\dfrac{3}{8}$$

$$\dfrac{7}{9} = \dfrac{7}{9}$$
$$-\dfrac{2}{3} = -\dfrac{6}{9}$$
$$\dfrac{1}{9}$$

Practice Set IV – 7
Subtract.

1. $\dfrac{3}{4}$

    $-\dfrac{3}{8}$

2. $\dfrac{5}{8}$

    $-\dfrac{1}{2}$

3. $\dfrac{1}{3}$

    $-\dfrac{1}{6}$

4. $\dfrac{1}{2}$

    $-\dfrac{3}{16}$

5. $\dfrac{15}{32}$

    $-\dfrac{1}{4}$

6. $\dfrac{1}{16}$

    $-\dfrac{1}{32}$

7. $\dfrac{17}{20}$

    $-\dfrac{1}{2}$

8. $\dfrac{9}{15}$

    $-\dfrac{1}{3}$

9. $\dfrac{11}{10}$

    $-\dfrac{1}{2}$

10. $\dfrac{16}{12}$

    $-\dfrac{1}{2}$

11. $\dfrac{12}{10}$

    $-\dfrac{1}{5}$

12. $\dfrac{12}{9}$

    $-\dfrac{1}{3}$

Subtracting Mixed Numbers

Subtract mixed numbers just as you added them — subtract the fractions, then subtract the whole numbers.

Example:

$$11\frac{5}{6} = 11\frac{10}{12}$$ Determine the LCD and convert the fractions

$$-3\frac{3}{4} = -3\frac{9}{12}$$ $$\frac{10}{12} - \frac{9}{12} = \frac{1}{12}$$

$$8\frac{1}{12}$$ and
$$11 - 3 = 8$$

Practice Set IV – 8

Subtract these mixed numbers. Be sure to reduce to lowest terms where possible.

1. $7\frac{5}{8}$
   $-4\frac{1}{4}$

2. $9\frac{5}{8}$
   $-5\frac{1}{2}$

3. $15\frac{3}{4}$
   $-11\frac{1}{2}$

4. $8\frac{3}{4}$
   $-5\frac{5}{8}$

5. $13\frac{11}{18}$
   $-12\frac{4}{9}$

6. $10\frac{2}{5}$
   $-3\frac{1}{4}$

7. $9\frac{3}{4}$
   $-\frac{2}{3}$

8. $62\frac{7}{10}$
   $-50\frac{7}{20}$

9. $6\frac{2}{3}$
   $-3\frac{1}{5}$

10. $14\frac{1}{2}$
    $-2\frac{1}{4}$

Subtracting Mixed Numbers where the Subtrahend Is a Larger Fraction

Example:

$$2\frac{1}{4}$$ Minuend - the number from which another is being subtracted

$$-\frac{3}{4}$$ Subtrahend - the number which is subtracted

Note that we wish to subtract $\frac{3}{4}$ from $\frac{1}{4}$. But $\frac{3}{4}$ is larger than $\frac{1}{4}$.

This procedure can only be completed by "borrowing". Borrow a whole number (1), change it into a fraction and add it to the minuend; then subtract.

Example: Borrow one from the two, convert to a fraction ($1 = \frac{4}{4}$), then subtract. Reduce if possible.

$$
\begin{array}{llll}
2\frac{1}{4} & = 1 + 1\frac{1}{4} & = 1 + \frac{4}{4} + \frac{1}{4} & = 1\frac{5}{4} \\
-\frac{3}{4} & = -\frac{3}{4} & = -\frac{3}{4} & = -\frac{3}{4} \\
& & & 1\frac{2}{4} = 1\frac{1}{2}
\end{array}
$$

Here is the same problem done another way and using a short cut.

$^{1}\cancel{2}\frac{1}{4}$ borrow 1(whole unit) from the 2

$-\frac{3}{4}$

_____

$^{1}\cancel{2}\frac{\overset{5}{\cancel{1}}}{4}$ add the numerator and denominator
together creating a new numerator

$-\frac{3}{4}$

_____

$1\frac{5}{4}$ this is the new
minuend

$-\frac{3}{4}$

_____

$1\frac{2}{4} = 1\frac{1}{2}$ subtract and
reduce

In practical terms, all you have to remember is to add the numerator and denominator (as in the first example) after you borrow. This works (as shown in detail in the second example) because any number over itself (that is, any time the numerator and denominator are the same) is equal to one. So if you borrow one whole number it will equal the same number of parts in which the fraction is represented.

If unlike denominators are represented, first determine the common denominator, then borrow and subtract. Here's an *example ...*

$$3\frac{1}{5}$$ determine the LCD $$3\frac{3}{15}$$ borrow $$2\cancel{3}\frac{18}{15}$$ Add the numerator and denominator $$2\frac{18}{15}$$

$$-1\frac{2}{3}$$ $$-1\frac{10}{15}$$ $$-1\frac{10}{15}$$ $$-1\frac{10}{15}$$ Subtract

$$1\frac{8}{15}$$

Practice Set IV – 9

Subtract the following mixed numbers:

1. $3\frac{2}{5}$ **2.** $4\frac{3}{4}$ **3.** $2\frac{1}{3}$ **4.** $1\frac{3}{4}$ **5.** $2\frac{3}{11}$

    $-2\frac{2}{3}$ $-1\frac{7}{8}$ $-\frac{5}{6}$ $-\frac{7}{8}$ $-\frac{7}{22}$

6. 16 **7.** 8 **8.** $1\frac{4}{9}$ **9.** $1\frac{9}{20}$ **10.** 9

   $-\frac{1}{2}$ $-\frac{4}{5}$ $-\frac{13}{18}$ $-\frac{4}{5}$ $-\frac{9}{16}$

Subtracting Improper Fractions

Except for the operation (subtraction), the techniques for subtracting are the same as for addition of improper fractions.

Examples:

(i) $\dfrac{11}{8}$

$-\dfrac{9}{8}$

$\dfrac{2}{8} = \dfrac{1}{4}$

(ii) $\dfrac{16}{4} = \dfrac{32}{8}$ Determine the LCD

                                Subtract

$-\dfrac{3}{8} = -\dfrac{3}{8}$ Convert to mixed number; reduce if necessary

$\dfrac{29}{8} = 3\dfrac{5}{8}$

Practice Set IV – 10
Subtract the following:

1. $\dfrac{11}{9}$

$-\dfrac{10}{9}$

2. $\dfrac{11}{9}$

$-\dfrac{4}{18}$

3. $\dfrac{5}{4}$

$-\dfrac{6}{5}$

4. $\dfrac{6}{5}$

$-\dfrac{7}{6}$

5. $\dfrac{51}{18}$

$-\dfrac{1}{9}$

Practice Set IV – Chapter Review
Solve each of the following:

1. $\dfrac{11}{17} + \dfrac{8}{34} =$

2. $1\dfrac{11}{17} - \dfrac{8}{34} =$

3. $\dfrac{1}{8} + \dfrac{1}{16} + \dfrac{3}{2} =$

4. $4\dfrac{1}{9} + 6\dfrac{11}{18} + 9\dfrac{1}{3} =$

5. $\dfrac{6}{8} - \dfrac{3}{5} =$

6. $4\dfrac{1}{8} - 1\dfrac{5}{7} =$

7. $1\dfrac{1}{2} + 2\dfrac{2}{3} + 3\dfrac{3}{4} + 4\dfrac{4}{5} =$

8. $4\dfrac{3}{4} - 3\dfrac{4}{5} =$

9. $4\dfrac{7}{8} - 2\dfrac{8}{9} =$

10. $6\dfrac{2}{3} - \dfrac{3}{4} =$

11. $1\dfrac{16}{17} - \dfrac{32}{34} =$

12. $\dfrac{7}{8} - \dfrac{2}{3} =$

13. $14\dfrac{5}{12} - 6\dfrac{9}{10} =$

14. $8\dfrac{3}{5} - \dfrac{7}{10} =$

15. $1\dfrac{5}{24} - \dfrac{1}{4} =$

16. $\dfrac{2}{3} - \dfrac{2}{6} =$

17. $1\dfrac{4}{9} - \dfrac{5}{18} =$

18. $4\dfrac{1}{3} - \dfrac{4}{9} =$

19. $4\dfrac{2}{7} + \dfrac{1}{2} =$

20. $8 - \dfrac{4}{9} =$

21. $18\dfrac{1}{24} + 1\dfrac{7}{8} =$

22. $\dfrac{1}{3} - \dfrac{1}{8} =$

23. $\dfrac{4}{16} - \dfrac{1}{4} =$

24. $7\dfrac{1}{4} + \dfrac{2}{3} =$

Chapter 5
Addition and Subtraction of Decimal Fractions

In the first few chapters we studied the four operations of common fractions. Now we study a different fraction that is very important and has everyday applications in the clinic and at the lab. The new fraction to be studied in this section is the decimal fraction. A *decimal fraction* may be considered a common fraction whose denominator is 10 (or some power of 10), such as denominators of 100, 1,000 and so on.

Examples:

$\dfrac{3}{10}$ can be written 0.3

$\dfrac{21}{100}$ can be written 0.21

$\dfrac{297}{1000}$ can be written 0.297

It is conventional to use a zero as the ones placeholder before the decimal to avoid any confusion and to point out that a decimal fraction follows.

Decimal Point	Tenths	Hundredths	Thousandths	Ten-Thousandths	Hundred-Thousandths
•					

All numbers to the left of the decimal point are *whole numbers*.

In the chart, notice that one place to the right of the decimal point is tenths; two places to the right of the decimal point is hundredths, three places thousandths, and so forth. When reading the decimal point we say "and".

Example: 2.57   is read   two *and* fifty-seven hundredths

An alternate method involves the words "decimal" or "point" and read the numerals as:

2.57 reads as two point five seven   or   two decimal fifty-seven

When writing (or reading) decimals of small values, less than one for example, zeros are placed between the decimal point and the number in the decimal (if necessary).

Examples: seven hundredths is written   0.07
                      nine thousandths   0.009

Practice Set V – 1

Write the following as decimal fractions.

1. nine tenths =

2. three tenths =

3. twenty-five hundredths =

4. nine ten-thousandths =

5. twelve thousandths =

6. twenty-two thousandths of an inch =

7. five tenths feet =

8. thirty-two thousandths =

Remember, decimals are really fractions, or parts, of a whole. We often use decimal representation instead of common fractions because decimal fractions can be simpler since they're based on powers of ten. We can easily change common fractions to decimal fractions by dividing the numerator by the denominator.

Example: Change $\dfrac{5}{8}$ to a decimal fraction.

$$\begin{array}{r} 0.625 \\ 8\overline{)5.000} \end{array}$$

Divide 5 by 8. Since 8 does not evenly divide into 5, we place the decimal point after the 5 (in the dividend), and immediately above that in the answer (the quotient). Annex zeros to the dividend and complete the division.

To convert a mixed number to a decimal, keep the whole number and convert the fractional part to a decimal as in the previous example.

$$1\frac{3}{4} \ = \ 1.75 \qquad \text{since} \quad 4\overline{)3.00}^{\,0.75}$$

Practice Set V – 2

Change the following common fractions to decimal fractions.

1. $\dfrac{11}{64}$

2. $\dfrac{3}{32}$

3. $\dfrac{5}{8}$

4. $\dfrac{5}{16}$

5. $\dfrac{1}{4}$

6. $\dfrac{1}{8}$

7. $\dfrac{5}{64}$

8. $\dfrac{1}{2}$

9. $1\dfrac{3}{8}$

10. $1\dfrac{7}{16}$

11. $\dfrac{3}{4}$

12. $\dfrac{7}{8}$

13. $2\dfrac{5}{8}$

14. $\dfrac{3}{80}$

15. $1\dfrac{9}{64}$

To change decimal fractions to common fractions:

    Example: change .45 to a common fraction.

$$.45 = \frac{45}{100} = \frac{9}{20} \text{ (reduced)}$$

decimal fraction   common fractions

Write the decimal, without the decimal point, over the appropriate tens units. Here, since the decimal is 45 hundredths, write 45 over 100.

Tip: count the decimal places and that indicates the number of zeros for the denominator.

Examples: (i) $0.456 = \dfrac{456}{1000}$ (ii) $0.0076 = \dfrac{76}{10,000}$

                  three decimal places, thus   four decimal places, thus
                  three zeros   four zeros

Practice Set V – 3

    Change each of the following to common fractions and reduce to lowest terms.

1. 0.06   **2.** 0.250   **3.** 0.495   **4.** 0.33   **5.** 0.630

6. 0.009   **7.** 0.3   **8.** 0.3755   **9.** 1.188   **10.** 0.40

Rounding Decimals

Sometimes, it is necessary to express an answer correct to the nearest hundredth or to the nearest thousandth, for example. After finding the solution, the answer may be rewritten with as many decimal places as are required to bring it to the degree of accuracy determined by the problem. This process is known as rounding off a number. *Rounding off* means expressing a decimal with fewer digits. The answer should be determined to one more place than the accuracy calls for, then *rounded* as indicated by that digit. Round to the nearest hundredth means the answer should have two decimal places. Thus, the answer should be carried to three places and the result rounded off to two places. If the digit to the right of the place you are rounding is 5 or more, drop it and add one to the digit in the place you are rounding. If the digit is less than 5, drop it and do not change digit in the place you are rounding.

Example: Round 0.671 to the nearest hundredth. Since the third decimal place (thousandths) is a 1, drop that and do not change the preceding digit (the 7) – the answer is then 0.67.

Round 0.876 to the nearest hundredth.

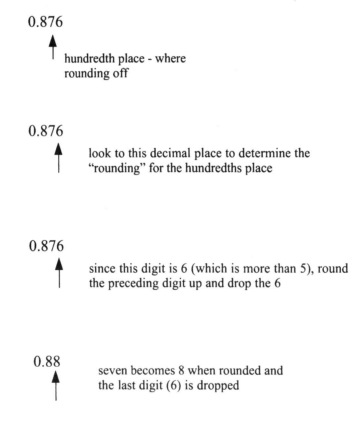

0.876

   hundredth place - where
   rounding off

0.876

   look to this decimal place to determine the
   "rounding" for the hundredths place

0.876

   since this digit is 6 (which is more than 5), round
   the preceding digit up and drop the 6

0.88

   seven becomes 8 when rounded and
   the last digit (6) is dropped

0.876 rounded to the nearest hundredth is 0.88

You try it! Round 0.7536 to the nearest thousandth.   *(answer: 0.754)*

Practice Set V – 4

Round each of the following to the nearest thousandth.

1. 0.8731   **2.** 0.7899   **3.** 0.7777

4. 0.6312   **5.** 0 .6214   **6.** 0.7325

Round each of the following to the nearest hundredth.

7. 0.654   **8.** 0.667   **9.** 0.372

10. 0.982   **11.** 0.427   **12.** 0.635

Round to the indicated (by underline) place.

13. 5<u>8</u>9   **14.** 0.003<u>2</u>9   **15.** 17<u>5</u>9

16. 0.<u>8</u>428   **17.** 1<u>6</u>07   **18.** 0.8<u>5</u>49

19. 19<u>0</u>5   **20.** 0.<u>0</u>02   **21.** 10<u>6</u>6

22. 1.9<u>8</u>08   **23.** <u>5</u>1   **24.** 4.<u>5</u>49

25. 14<u>3</u>2   **26.** 1.4<u>3</u>2   **27.** 876<u>9</u>29

Addition of Decimals

You already know how to add dollars and cents. Add all decimals the same way! The key to remember is to align the decimal points in a column. Add just as you would for whole numbers, placing the decimal point in the answer directly below the column of decimal points.

Example: Add.   6.25 + 21.021 + 873.0725 + 647

        6.25
        21.021
        873.0725
        647.   a common error involves "forgetting" that the decimal in a
                                        whole number belongs at the right end of that number

Some students like to even the columns using zeros in those numbers with fewer places so everything "lines up". Like this:

                6.2500
                21.0210
                873.0725
                647.0000
                ————————
                1547.3435

Practice Set V – 5

Add the following.

1. 0.008, 20, 0.6, 4.5   **2.** 0.03, 0.3, 4.12, 30

3. 10, 0.0615, 1.2   **4.** 52.2, 0.06, 0.0008, 2000

5. 0.005, 2.5, 1.1

6. 0.006, 5, 0.32, 0.08

7. 0.05, 10.256, 12.2

8. 0.09, 10, 4.8, 1000

9. 0.05, 0.006, 0.032, 0.0003

10. 2.5, 1.98, 100, 0.8

11. 1.2, 1.5, 0.03, 15

12. 0.15, 0.4, 0.048, 6

13. 0.8, 1.5, 0.5

14. 0.64, 8, 0.06, 0.3

Subtraction of Decimals

Subtraction of decimals in done in the same manner. Align the decimal points, subtract, place the decimal in the answer directly in the same column place as each of the decimals. Again, you may add zeros so that all numbers align.

Example: subtract 15.275 from 32.63

$$
\begin{array}{r}
32.63 \\
-15.275 \\
\hline
17.355
\end{array}
\qquad
\begin{array}{r}
32.630 \\
-15.275 \\
\hline
17.355
\end{array}
$$

Practice Set V – 6

Subtract.

1. 92.12 minus 0.37

2. 1,000 minus 810.77

3. 11,246.51 minus 247.59

4. 53.36 minus 43.65

5. 0.0257 from 9.3126

6. 4.695 from 7.342

7. 0.079 from 0.1032

8. 0.65832 from 1

Chapter 6
Multiplication and Division of Decimal Fractions

Multiplication of Decimals

In the previous chapter you learned how to add and subtract with decimals. In this section, we learn how to multiply and divide with decimals.

When multiplying numbers, the result, or answer, is called the product. The numbers being multiplied are called factors.

Examples: $5 \times 15 = 75$ The product is 75. The factors are 5 and 15.

$$\frac{1}{2} \times \frac{2}{3} = \frac{2}{6} = \frac{1}{3}$$ The product is $1/3$. The factors are $1/2$ and $2/3$.

$0.3 \times 0.5 = .15$ The product is 0.15. The factors are 0.3 and 0.5.

In the examples shown, it doesn't matter if the numbers are whole numbers, common fractions, or decimal fractions – the answer is called the product in each case of multiplication.

When multiplying decimals, proceed as in multiplying whole numbers. The process is the same. The only change is placing the decimal point in the proper position in the resultant product. Count the number of decimal places in each of the numbers multiplied. Place the decimal to the right of the product, as if it was a whole number, and move the decimal point one place to the left for each decimal place in the factors.

Example:
$$\begin{array}{r} 5 \\ \times\, 0.12 \\ \hline \end{array}$$
How many decimal places are there? _____

Your answer should have two decimal places for the two places in the factor 0.12. In the product start with the rightmost digit and move two decimal places to the left:

$$
\begin{array}{r}
5 \\
\times\,0.12 \\
\hline
0.60
\end{array}
$$

5   There are no decimal places to the right of this whole number.

× 0.12   There are 2 decimal places in this factor.

0.60

The answer must have 2 decimal places.
Beginning at the far right, move 2 places
to the left and place the decimal.

Practice Set VI – 1

Determine the placement of the decimal point for each of the products shown.

1.	2.	3.	4.	5.
0.35	94	0.707	1.6	0.0638
× 4	× 0.4	× 0.2	× 40	× 0.78
140	376	1414	640	49764

Note: in number **5** the sum of the decimal points to be counted off is *six*. Yet the product has only five digits. In these cases, insert one or more zeros to the *left* of the product in order to have the required number of decimal places. The answer for (**5**) should be: 0.049764

Practice Set VI – 2

Multiply. Place the decimal point in the correct position in the product.

1. $17.5 \times 6 =$ **2.** $168 \times 0.321 =$ **3.** $4.8 \times 0.067 =$

4. $0.56 \times 0.83 =$ **5.** $63 \times 37.91 =$ **6.** $0.72 \times 0.095 =$

7. Multiply 0.2279 by 0.029

8. Multiply 6.85 by 81.2

9. $306.693 \times 2.61 =$

10. Find the product of 18.35 and 0.065

11. Wages for 29 hours of work at $ 5.12 per hour are ?

12. Find the cost of 212 bushels of corn at $ 3.08 per bushel.

13. Find the cost of 98 instruments at $5.88 each

14. How much is 32 quarts of milk at $1.19 a quart?

15. 18 dozen eggs at $ 1.55 per dozen is how much?

In the lab, you may need to multiply by 10 or 100 or 1000. These all represent multiples of ten. There is a short cut to multiplying by multiples of ten. For example, multiply 2.4 by 10, 100, and 1000.

$$2.4 \times 10 = 24$$
$$2.4 \times 100 = 240.0$$
$$2.4 \times 1000 = 2400.0$$

When 2.4 is multiplied by 10, How does the decimal place change in the product?

When multiplying a number by ten, move the decimal of that number one place to the right in the product. When multiplying by 1,000 the decimal point is moved three places to the right in the product.

Practice Set VI – 3

Multiply the following.

1. 3.6×10 **2.** 5.4×1000

3. 0.47×100 **4.** 9.61×100

5. 2.45×1000 **6.** 7.1×10

Division of Decimals

Now we learn how to divide using decimals. Recall that in multiplication the answer, or result is called the product. In division, the answer is called the quotient. The number that is being divided is called the dividend; and the number with which the dividend is divided is called the divisor.

Example:

$$\underset{divisor}{}\overline{)\underset{dividend}{}} \quad \overset{quotient}{}$$

$$\text{divisor} \longrightarrow 6\overline{)42} \quad \underset{\longleftarrow \text{ dividend}}{\overset{7 \ \longleftarrow \text{ quotient}}{}}$$

To divide a decimal by a whole number, simply divide and place the decimal point in the quotient directly above the decimal point in the dividend.

Examples:

$$16\overline{)6.4}^{\ .4} \qquad\qquad 22\overline{).88}^{\ .04} \qquad\qquad 13\overline{)26.}^{\ 2.}$$

Practice Set VI – 4
Divide. Round answers to 3 decimal places, if necessary.

1. $25\overline{)6.50}$ 2. $44\overline{)9.24}$ 3. $16\overline{).922}$

4. $14\overline{).42}$ 5. $12\overline{)2.64}$ 6. $25\overline{)1.75}$

7. $25\overline{)75.25}$ 8. $47\overline{)317.72}$ 9. $64\overline{)131.2}$

Suppose we wanted to divide a whole number by some decimal number. Such as: $0.16\overline{)32}$

The divisor is 0.16 and the dividend is 32. With division, the divisor must always be made into a whole number by moving the decimal place to the right. In this case, the decimal point is moved two places to the right. To complement this procedure, we must also then move the decimal place of the dividend two places to the right as well. Finally, place the decimal point in the quotient, the answer, directly above the new position in the dividend. Like this

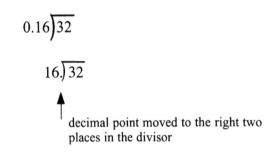

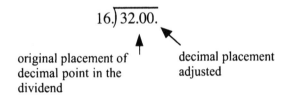

Finally, do the division: $16.\overline{)3200.}$ with quotient $200.$ The decimal in the quotient is directly above the decimal in the dividend.

Practice Set VI – 5

Divide. Round answer to thousandths (3 places), if necessary.

1. $1.2\overline{)36}$ 2. $1.3\overline{)650}$ 3. $0.5\overline{)75}$

4. $0.08\overline{)64}$ **5.** $0.9\overline{)72}$ **6.** $0.25\overline{)200}$

From (**6**), here is another look at that problem.

$.25\overline{)200}$ $= 200 \div .25$

$= 200 \div \dfrac{1}{4}$ since $0.25 = \dfrac{1}{4}$

$= 200 \times \dfrac{4}{1}$ as learned when dividing fractions

$= 800$

To divide a decimal by another decimal, move the decimal point of the divisor to the right until the divisor becomes a whole number. Then move the decimal point in the dividend the same number of places, annexing zeros if necessary. Next, place the decimal point in the quotient. Finally, divide as one would with whole numbers.

Example: $4.5 \div 0.15$

$$.15\overline{\smash{)}4.50.}^{30.}$$

The decimal point in the divisor and the dividend is moved two places to the right.

Practice Set VI – 6

Round answers to three decimal places, if necessary.

1. Divide 9801.9 by 0.9   **2.** Divide 892.5 by 7.0

3. Divide 58.32 by 1.8   **4.** Divide 17.28 by 0.12

5. Divide 5.12 by 0.08   **6.** Divide 3.43 by 0.7

7. Divide 306.72 by 0.8   **8.** Divide 793.1 by 0.07

9. Divide 100.1 by 0.001   **10.** Divide 795.07 by 4.3

11. $0.0075\overline{)0.6}$ **12.** $0.25\overline{)75.25}$

13. $4.7\overline{)317.72}$ **14.** $6.4\overline{)873.42}$

You have divided decimals into whole numbers, whole numbers into decimals, and decimals into decimals. Now practice placing the decimal point in the quotient.

Practice Set VI – 7

Location of decimal point

The answer for each of the following contains the digits 343. You must correctly place the decimal point in the answer, adding zeros where necessary. The first couple are done for you as examples. It is not necessary to actually do the division since every answer contains the given digits.

1. $124\overline{)42.532}$ with quotient $.343$

2. $124\overline{)425.32}$ with quotient 3.43

3. $1.24\overline{)42.532}$

4. $.124\overline{)425.32}$

5. $12.4\overline{)4253.2}$

6. $12.4\overline{).42532}$

7. $1.24\overline{)4253.2}$

8. $124\overline{).42532}$

9. $.124\overline{).42532}$

10. $12.4\overline{)4.2532}$

11. $1.24\overline{).042532}$

12. $12.4\overline{)42.532}$

13. $0.124\overline{)4253.2}$

14. $0.124\overline{).042532}$

15. $.00124\overline{).0042532}$

16. $.124\overline{).0042532}$

17. $1.24\overline{).0042532}$

18. $124\overline{).042532}$

Practice Set VI – 8 Review

Perform the indicated operation.

1. $\begin{array}{r} 0.315 \\ \times\,3.12 \\ \hline \end{array}$

2. $\begin{array}{r} 9.10 \\ \times\,9.1 \\ \hline \end{array}$

3. $\begin{array}{r} 56.7 \\ \times\,0.42 \\ \hline \end{array}$

4. $\begin{array}{r} 0.096 \\ \times\,7.8 \\ \hline \end{array}$

5. $\begin{array}{r} 357.1 \\ \times\,0.111 \\ \hline \end{array}$

6. $\begin{array}{r} 5.03 \\ \times\,0.9111 \\ \hline \end{array}$

7. $\begin{array}{r} 2.56 \\ \times\,0.48 \\ \hline \end{array}$

8. $\begin{array}{r} 600.73 \\ \times\,1.12 \\ \hline \end{array}$

9. $\begin{array}{r} 1.512 \\ \times\,1.34 \\ \hline \end{array}$

10. $\begin{array}{r} 2.432 \\ \times\,0.07 \\ \hline \end{array}$

11. $\begin{array}{r} 0.431 \\ \times\,0.32 \\ \hline \end{array}$

12. $\begin{array}{r} 7.62 \\ \times\,3.1 \\ \hline \end{array}$

13. $\begin{array}{r} 8.031 \\ \times\,1.34 \\ \hline \end{array}$

14. $\begin{array}{r} 1.213 \\ \times\,0.561 \\ \hline \end{array}$

15. $\begin{array}{r} 2.521 \\ \times\,6.21 \\ \hline \end{array}$

16. $\begin{array}{r} 7.36 \\ \times\,0.62 \\ \hline \end{array}$

17. 9.023
× 1.45
___

18. 3.123
× 0.654
___

19. 1.125
× 5.11
___

20. 6.37
× 0.22
___

21. 2.5
× 2.1
___

22. 9.16
× 1.72
___

23. 15.4
× 1.2
___

24. 0.0786
× 2.4
___

25. 14.807
× 4.1
___

26. 89.7
× 5.3
___

27. 15.4
× 70
___

28. 98.23
× 100
___

29. 14.887
× 0.1
___

30. 22.73
× 0.01
___

31. 17.1
× 0.001
___

32. 12.89
× 0.0001
___

Divide. Round answers to thousandths, if necessary.

1. $1.8 \div 0.002$

2. $1.616 \div 0.77$

3. $76.4 \div 38.2$

4. $98.65 \div 13.1$

5. $3.6503 \div 1.25$

6. $9.9 \div 3.3$

7. $0.567 \div 14$

8. $3.693 \div 0.03$

9. $50.25 \div 0.5$

10. $200 \div 2.5$

11. $5.40 \div 0.6$

12. $24.57 \div 2.7$

13. $7.5 \div 1.5$

14. $0.006 \div 0.003$

15. $84.84 \div 4.2$

16. $200 \div 2.8$ **17.** $42.63 \div 100$ **18.** $3.655 \div 10$

19. $98.3525 \div 1000$ **20.** $8.359 \div 0.1$ **21.** $8.359 \div 0.01$

22. $8.359 \div 0.001$ **23.** $5.40 \div 0.01$ **24.** $24.56 \div 0.03$

Often, while doing lab work, a need arises to divide by ten, one hundred, 1000, one tenth, one hundredth, or so on. As when multiplying by powers of ten, dividing by powers of ten also can be short cut.

Example: Divide 2.4 by each of the following . . .

$2.4 \div 10 = .24$ $2.4 \div 0.1 = 24$

$2.4 \div 100 = .024$ $2.4 \div 0.01 = 240$

$2.4 \div 1000 = .0024$ $2.4 \div 0.001 = 2400$

In the example above, when we divided 2.4 by 10, how did the decimal point change?

You noticed that the decimal point moved one place to the left in the quotient when dividing by ten. When we divided by 0.001 ($^1/_{1000}$) the decimal point moved three places to the *right* in the quotient. So, when dividing by whole number multiples of ten, the decimal point moves one place left in the quotient for each zero in the divisor. On the other hand, division by multiples of ten less than one, like $^1/10$ or $^1/_{100}$, the decimal point is adjusted right according to the number of decimal places in the divisor.

Practice Set VI – 9

Divide. Practice using the rules for division by powers of 10.

1. $0.01\overline{)314.2}$

2. $1000\overline{)314.2}$

3. $10\overline{)314.2}$

4. $0.001\overline{)3.142}$

5. $100\overline{)31.42}$

6. $0.0001\overline{)314.2}$

7. 314.2 divided *by* 10,000

8. 0.3142 divided by 0.1

9. 100,000 divided *into* 314.2

10. 0.000001 divided into 3.142

The following practice set involves multiplying and dividing by powers of ten. This relationship will be further explored with scientific notation later in this chapter. Try using some short cut method when possible.

Practice Set VI – 10 Perform the indicated operation relocating the decimal point as indicated.

	Multiply	*Divide*
1.	$231 \times 10 =$	$231 \div 10 =$
2.	2001×0.0001	$2001 \div 0.0001$
3.	48.236×1000	$48.236 \div 1000$
4.	2.310×0.01	$2.310 \div 0.01$
5.	4.691×100	$4.691 \div 100$
6.	96.39×1000	$96.39 \div 1000$

7. 856.9×0.0001 $856.9 \div 0.0001$

8. 9.8751×0.001 $9.8751 \div 0.001$

9. 18.754×10 $18.754 \div 10$

10. 910.4×100 $910.4 \div 100$

Scientific Notation

To convert to scientific notation from a decimal

- based on powers of ten
- Format: $N \times 10^x$ where $1 \leq N < 10$ and x is any integer

Easy to convert by simply moving the decimal point:

- for a number greater than one (1)

⟵————————— move the decimal point the required "steps" to the Left
The number of steps represents x and x is positive.

- for a number less than 1

—————————⟶ move the decimal point the required steps to the Right. The number of steps represents x and x is negative.

Here's how it works ...

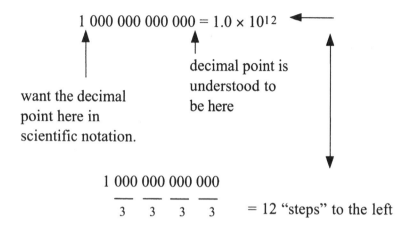

1 000 000 000 000 = 1.0×10^{12}

want the decimal point here in scientific notation.

decimal point is understood to be here

1 000 000 000 000

3   3   3   3   = 12 "steps" to the left

... this gives the desired **N** such that **N** is (at least) 1.0 and the power of ten corresponds to the number of places ("steps") taken!

Examples:

$1000 = 1.0 \times 10^3$ $1520 = 1.52 \times 10^3$ $0.003 = 3 \times 10^{-3}$

$0.00415 = 4.15 \times 10^{-3}$ $10004000 = 1.0004 \times 10^7$

$0.0000045 = 4.5 \times 10^{-6}$ $1\ 000\ 000\ 000\ 000\ 000 = 1.0 \times 10^{15}$

To convert to a decimal from scientific notation

The sign (positive/negative) of the exponent of ten (10^x) determines the direction to move when converting from scientific notation to standard numbers.

- if the sign of the exponent is negative move the decimal that many places left

- if the sign of the exponent is positive, move the decimal point to the right

Examples:

$1.4 \times 10^3 = 1400$ $\qquad$ $2.0 \times 10^5 = 200000$ $\qquad$ $3.1 \times 10^{-4} = 0.00031$

$9.5 \times 10^{-7} = 0.00000095$ $\qquad$ $4.3 \times 10^2 = 430$

$4.5 \times 10^{-6} = 0.0000045$

$\qquad$ move decimal point 6 places to the left (since exponent is *negative*)

You may have noticed that scientific notation with negative exponents indicate decimal numbers less than one. Positive exponents in scientific notation indicate numbers greater than, or equal to, one. Furthermore, any number times one remains the same.

Practice Set VI – 11

Express each of the following in scientific notation.

1. 100,000 $\qquad$ **2.** 100 $\qquad$ **3.** 1,000,000

4. 0.0001 $\qquad$ **5.** 0.01 $\qquad$ **6.** 0.00000001

7. 0.0000000001 $\qquad$ **8.** 0.000001 $\qquad$ **9.** 1000

10. 10,000,000

Rewrite each of the following from scientific notation to whole number or decimal form.

11. 10^6 or 1×10^6 **12.** 10^4 or 1×10^4 **13.** 10^3 or 1×10^3

14. 10^7 **15.** 10^{-3} **16.** 10^{-5}

17. 10^{-2} **18.** 10^{-6} **19.** 10^2

Practice Set VI – 12

Convert to/from scientific notation, as appropriate.

1. 2×10^4 **2.** 8.4×10^6

3. 0.33×10^{-2} **4.** 0.33×10^2

5. 8.47×10^{-8} **6.** 0.00035

7. 0.000839 **8.** 10857

9. 87.69×10^8 **10.** 4.235×10^{-4}

11. 6.798×10^{-7}

12. 246810

13. 0.00357

14. 8.276×10^{-5}

15. 7.5×10^{-6}

16. 15×10^{-6}

17. 4×10^{7}

18. 0.0000436

19. 45789

20. 257

21. 8324.67

22. 2.69×10^{4}

23. 0.00357

24. 0.00005

25. 0.00001

Fraction Review

Add and reduce to lowest terms.

1. $2\frac{2}{9}$
    $1\frac{1}{27}$
    $\frac{6}{18}$
    $+\frac{1}{3}$

2. $5\frac{1}{8}$
    $2\frac{3}{64}$
    $\frac{5}{24}$
    $+3\frac{1}{4}$

3. $6\frac{1}{4}$
    $\frac{5}{6}$
    $12\frac{5}{8}$
    $+\frac{12}{32}$

4. $5\frac{6}{8}$
    $6\frac{1}{4}$
    $12\frac{1}{6}$
    $+1\frac{3}{8}$

5. $\frac{7}{8}$
    $\frac{3}{4}$
    $+\frac{9}{10}$

Convert to mixed or whole numbers. Reduce and express in lowest terms.

6. $\frac{20}{5} =$

7. $\frac{16}{5} =$

8. $\frac{50}{6} =$

9. $\frac{13}{12} =$

10. $\frac{36}{12} =$

11. $\frac{56}{6} =$

12. $\frac{42}{3} =$

13. $\frac{19}{4} =$

14. $\frac{72}{8} =$

15. $\frac{7}{2} =$

Multiply. Reduce to lowest terms.

16. $\dfrac{2}{3} \times \dfrac{5}{12} =$

17. $1\dfrac{1}{4} \times 8\dfrac{1}{5} =$

18. $2\dfrac{1}{2} \times 3\dfrac{1}{4} \times 8\dfrac{4}{5} =$

19. $\dfrac{7}{9} \times \dfrac{1}{5} =$

20. $2\dfrac{3}{5} \times 4\dfrac{1}{5} =$

21. $\dfrac{24}{25} \times \dfrac{11}{20} =$

22. $1\dfrac{3}{4} \times 2\dfrac{3}{4} =$

23. $3\dfrac{3}{4} \times 1\dfrac{3}{5} \times 2\dfrac{4}{5} =$

24. $\dfrac{1}{3} \times 4\dfrac{1}{2} =$

25. $\dfrac{5}{12} \times \dfrac{2}{3} =$

26. $3\dfrac{1}{6} \times 6\dfrac{2}{3} =$

27. $\dfrac{3}{4} \times \dfrac{2}{5} =$

28. $2\dfrac{1}{6} \times 4\dfrac{7}{8} =$

29. $\dfrac{3}{5} \times \dfrac{3}{2} =$

30. $8\dfrac{2}{5} \times 2\dfrac{3}{5} =$

31. $\dfrac{5}{8} \times \dfrac{4}{5} =$

32. $2\dfrac{1}{3} \times 3\dfrac{3}{5} =$

33. $12\dfrac{1}{2} \times 17\dfrac{1}{3} \times 3\dfrac{3}{4} =$

Subtract and reduce to lowest terms.

34.
$$\begin{array}{r} \dfrac{7}{8} \\[2mm] -\dfrac{1}{4} \\[1mm] \hline \end{array}$$

35.
$$\begin{array}{r} 5\dfrac{4}{5} \\[2mm] -2\dfrac{3}{5} \\[1mm] \hline \end{array}$$

36.
$$\begin{array}{r} 12\dfrac{1}{2} \\[2mm] -2\dfrac{1}{6} \\[1mm] \hline \end{array}$$

37.
$$\begin{array}{r} \dfrac{9}{10} \\[2mm] -\dfrac{3}{5} \\[1mm] \hline \end{array}$$

38.
$$\begin{array}{r} 15\dfrac{2}{3} \\[2mm] -3\dfrac{2}{3} \\[1mm] \hline \end{array}$$

39.
$$\begin{array}{r} \dfrac{7}{10} \\[2mm] -\dfrac{2}{5} \\[1mm] \hline \end{array}$$

40.
$$\begin{array}{r} \dfrac{11}{16} \\[2mm] -\dfrac{1}{2} \\[1mm] \hline \end{array}$$

41.
$$\begin{array}{r} 19\dfrac{1}{2} \\[2mm] -11\dfrac{1}{4} \\[1mm] \hline \end{array}$$

42.
$$\begin{array}{r} 61\dfrac{2}{3} \\[2mm] -2\dfrac{4}{5} \\[1mm] \hline \end{array}$$

43.
$$\begin{array}{r} 1\dfrac{1}{2} \\[2mm] -\dfrac{3}{4} \\[1mm] \hline \end{array}$$

Divide. Reduce to lowest terms.

44. $8\dfrac{5}{8} \div \dfrac{1}{50} =$

45. $\dfrac{4}{75} \div \dfrac{7}{25} =$

46. $12\dfrac{4}{5} \div 5\dfrac{1}{2} =$

47. $25\dfrac{1}{2} \div 7\dfrac{3}{4} =$

48. $\dfrac{3}{20} \div \dfrac{1}{2} =$

49. $\dfrac{4}{25} \div \dfrac{8}{25} =$

50. $190\dfrac{3}{4} \div 2\dfrac{5}{8} =$

51. $4\dfrac{1}{5} \div 2\dfrac{9}{10} =$

52. $1\dfrac{1}{2} \div \dfrac{3}{4} =$

Unit II

Chapter 7
Percentage

There is a need to know how to compute percentage both in business and industry. Many handbooks, manuals, and catalogs make references to percents. The sign, or symbol, for percent is %. Percent means *per hundred.* Per means divide, and cent refers to 100. Thus, percent means something divided by 100. 40% is read forty percent and indicates 40 hundredths or 40 parts out of 100.

Changing Percent to a Number

Math operations involving percentages, such as multiplication and division, cannot be computed in the form using the symbol %. We must change the percent into a decimal or common fraction. Since percent means hundredths, we can change percent into a decimal. Recall that hundred*ths* is two (decimal) places to the right of the decimal point. In a whole number, the decimal is understood to be at the rightmost place of the number.

Examples: 8 is the same as 8.0

                    97 is the same as 97.0

When multiplying a number by 100, we learned to move the decimal point two places to the right. If dividing by 100, move the decimal two places to the left. Percent means divide by 100. Therefore, to change a percent to a decimal drop the % sign and move the decimal two places to the left.

Examples: 81% = 0.81

                    96% = 0.96

                    5%   = 0.05

                    112% = 1.12

Practice Set VII – 1

Change the following % to decimals.

1. 15%   **2.** 1%   **3.** 94.3%

4. 33%   **5.** 9%   **6.** 100%

7. 40%   **8.** 125%   **9.** 5%

To change a decimal to a percent move the decimal point two places to the right and append the percent sign, %.

Examples: 0.12 = 12%

                   0.07 = 7%

                   1.19 = 119%

Practice Set VII – 2

Change the following decimals to percent:

                   1. 0.10   **2.** 6.3   **3.** 0.9

                   4. 0.12   **5.** 0.762   **6.** .375

                   7. 0.125   **8.** 0.875   **9.** .085

                   10. 0.09   **11.** 2.25   **12.** 0.1

To change from a percent to a common fraction requires expressing the value of the percent as a fraction rather than a decimal. To do this, use the value of the percent as the numerator and 100 as the denominator. Reduce as necessary.

Examples: $21\% = \dfrac{21}{100}$ $\qquad$ $40\% = \dfrac{40}{100} = \dfrac{2}{5}$ $\qquad$ $75\% = \dfrac{75}{100} = \dfrac{3}{4}$

Practice Set VII – 3

Change the given percents to common fractions. Be sure to reduce.

1. 60% $\qquad\qquad$ **2.** 10% $\qquad\qquad$ **3.** 110%

4. 50% $\qquad\qquad$ **5.** 8% $\qquad\qquad$ **6.** 90%

To change any fraction to percent, first change the fraction to a decimal by dividing the denominator into the numerator. Then change the resulting decimal to a percent as previously discussed. *(See Practice Set VII – 2.)*

Examples: $\quad$ Change $\dfrac{1}{2}$ to percent $\qquad 2\overline{)1.0}^{\,.5} = 0.5 = 50\%$

$\qquad\qquad\qquad$ Write $3/8$ as a percent $\qquad \dfrac{3}{8} = 8\overline{)3.000}^{\,.375} = 0.375 = 37.5\%$

Practice Set VII – 4

Change the following fractions to percents. If necessary, round to the nearest tenth of a percent.

1. $\dfrac{1}{4}$

2. $\dfrac{1}{12}$

3. $\dfrac{5}{6}$

4. $\dfrac{3}{5}$

5. $\dfrac{3}{16}$

6. $\dfrac{1}{5}$

7. $\dfrac{7}{10}$

8. $\dfrac{7}{8}$

Practice Set VII – 5

Express each of the following percents as a decimal.

1. 12.5%

2. 8.5%

3. 57.11%

4. 6.25%

5. 9.5%

6. 190%

Express each of the following decimals as a percent.

7. 0.33   **8.** 0.3633   **9.** 0.987

10. 0.63   **11.** 0.11   **12.** 16.375

Express each of the following fractions to the nearest tenth of a percent.

13. $\dfrac{1}{8}$ **14.** $\dfrac{5}{8}$ **15.** $\dfrac{1}{7}$

16. $\dfrac{4}{7}$ **17.** $\dfrac{1}{9}$ **18.** $\dfrac{5}{9}$

19. $\dfrac{1}{11}$ **20.** $\dfrac{7}{11}$

Express each of the following percents as a common fraction and reduce to lowest terms where necessary.

Examples: $5\% = \dfrac{5}{100} = \dfrac{1}{20}$ Or, working with the decimal form $5\% = .05 = \dfrac{5}{100} = \dfrac{1}{20}$

$$12.5\% = .125 = \dfrac{125}{1000} = \dfrac{1}{8}$$

21. 2%   **22.** 72%   **23.** 20%

24. 40%   **25.** 32%   **26.** 48%

27. 38.5%   **28.** 1.75%

Complete the following chart. Express each of the following as a percent, as a decimal and/or a fraction or mixed number.

	Fraction	Decimal	Percent
29.			8%
30.			7.5%
31.		0.925	
32.			66.7%
33.	$\frac{3}{7}$		
34.		0.125	
35.		650.00	
36.	$\frac{9}{16}$		
37.			125%
38.	$\frac{11}{42}$		
39.		0.333	
40.	$3\frac{5}{8}$		
41.	$1\frac{5}{9}$		
42.			3.25%

Now that we know the mechanics of changing percents to decimals and fractions and back again, we can use that knowledge to solve problems involving percentages. To find the percent of a given number use the following guidelines:

- Convert the percent to either a fractional or decimal equivalent.
- Multiply the given number by this equivalent.
- Label answer with appropriate unit of measure.

Examples: *(i)*   Find 16% of 1218 millimeters.

Step 1:   Change 16% to a decimal   16% = .16

Step 2:   Multiply

1218
×.16
194.88

Step 3:   Label answer   194.88 millimeters is 16% of 1218 ml *(ii)* Follow the same steps when the percent is a mixed number.

Find 6 $^1/_4$ % of 782 hours

Step 1: 6 $^1/_4$ % = 6.25% = 0.0625

Step 2:

$$\begin{array}{r} 782 \\ \times .0625 \\ \hline 48.8750 \end{array}$$

Step 3: 48.875 hours

Here is one way to think about percentage problems. Consider –

x percent   of n is y

Of means "times" and *is* means "equals". *x percent* must be a decimal to perform any arithmetic. *n* generally is the total, or original amount. *y* is the part of the total, or the amount of increase, or the amount of decrease. You will always know, or be able to determine, two of these three parts.

A way to remember this is to make a sentence as a pneumonic device. For example, "What percent of something is this?"

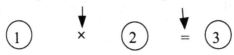

$$x\% \quad \text{of} \quad n \quad \text{is} \quad y$$

What percent of something is this?

$$\textcircled{1} \quad \times \quad \textcircled{2} \quad = \quad \textcircled{3}$$

	①	×	②	=	③	
(1) 35% of 52 is ? In this case, the model is	35%	×	52	=	???	change 35% to a decimal and multiply (= 18.2)
(2) What percent of 52 is 18.2?	???	×	52	=	18.2	divide 18.2 by 52; change the resultant decimal to percent (.35 = 35%)
(3) 35% of what is 18.2?	35%	×	???	=	18.2	divide 18.2 by 0.35 to get 52

Practice Set VII – 6

Solve each of the following. Round answer to three places, if necessary.

1. 5% of 1000

2. 20% of 555

3. 50% of 1000

4. 12.5% of 480

5. 6.25% of 800

6. 33.3% of 500

7. 10% of 750

8. 20% of 500

9. 25% of 1200

10. 37.5% of 1200

11. 16.67% of 180

12. 40% of 1200

Word problems are practical situations where various mathematical procedures are used. The following is an example of percentage word problems.

Example:

       A clinic has 43,560 square feet of floor space. An expansion is planned that will increase the floor space 25%. (a) Find the amount of floor space that is being added. (b) Find the total floor space after the addition.

$$\begin{array}{r} 43,560 \\ \times\, 0.25 \\ \hline 10,890.00 \end{array}$$ (a) 25% of 43,560 is added floor space: 10,890 sq. ft.

      (b) 43,560 sq. ft. + 10,890 sq. ft. = 54, 450 sq. ft.

      floor space + increased space = total floor space after addition

Practice Set VII – 7

    Solve the following word problems. Round to two places, if necessary.

1. One doctor figured a procedure at a cost of $940.00. A second doctor quoted a price that was 25% less. What was the second price?

2. Seventy-five pounds of brass contains 45% zinc and the balance is copper. Determine the number of pounds of zinc.

3. A shipment of chemicals was billed at $548.00 but it was damaged in transit. An allowance of 15% was made for the damages. What is the net amount due?

4. A technician measured 500 ml of distilled water. Eighteen percent of the water was used in the lab. How much distilled water was left?

Determining what percent one number is of another

Example: 20 is what percent of 50   or written another way: 20 = ? % of 50

   y is *x* %   of   *n*

Write the numbers as a fraction. The number to be compared (20) is the numerator. The number with which it to be compared (50) is the denominator.

$$\text{Part} \longrightarrow \frac{20}{50} = \frac{2}{5}$$
$$\text{Total, or original} \longrightarrow$$

change the fraction to a decimal

$$5)\overline{2.0}^{.4}$$ change 0.4 to percent

0.4 = 40%   20 is 40% of 50.

20 is the part of the total 50. Divide the part by the total or original amount.

Example: In measuring 80 lbs. of chemicals, 1.6 pounds was lost by accident. What percent was lost?

1.6 = ? % of 80   Thus,   Part $\longrightarrow \dfrac{1.6}{80}$
            Total, or original $\longrightarrow$

Simplifying $80)\overline{1.60}^{.02}$ writing the decimal as a percent   0.02 = 2% was lost

Practice Set VII – 8

Solve the following problems. Round percents to nearest tenth percent.

1. 27 lbs. of lab chemicals were ordered, but 8 lbs. were lost in shipment. What percent was lost?

2. Given 125 lbs. of chemicals, 2.56 lbs. was lost. What percent was lost?

3. The lab had 11 lbs. of chemicals, 1.1 lbs. were lost. What percent loss is this?

4. Inspecting 50 bottles used for dispensing medication, 4 were found to be broken. What percent were broken?

5. In working 45 problems on a test, 7 were incorrect. What percent were incorrect?

6. After 11 days at work you missed a day. What percent of those 12 days total have you missed?

7. A man working for $6.40 per hour has his pay increased by 52 cents per hour. What percent increase did he receive?

8. John uses $2\,3/4$ pounds of cleaner from a canister containing 12 lbs. of cleaner. What percent of the cleaner was removed?

9. For a certain laboratory experiment, a resultant weighing 3.25 lbs. is obtained. If the total weight of the chemical components of the experiment were 4.59 lbs. , then the weight of the resultant is what percent of the components?

10. Raw materials for a certain type of hospital bed weigh 327 lbs. A finished bed weighs 288 lbs. What percent of the raw material is lost in manufacture?

Determining a new price when there is a percent change is common. This could be the result of a price increase due to inflation or a price decrease due to a discount. Either way, the procedures are similar.

Price Increase

1. Find the change by converting the percent to its decimal equivalent and multiplying by the price.
2. Add the increase in the price to the original price to find the new price.

Example: 9% increase in an object which originally cost $15.49

9% = 0.09   Use the decimal equivalent

x% of n is y

9% of 15.49 is

0.09 • 15.49=

$15.49	Original cost		$15.49	Original cost
× 0.09	Amount of increase		+ 1.39	Amount of increase
$1.3941 = $1.39			$16.88	Total new price

Price Decrease

1. Find the change by converting the percent to its decimal equivalent and multiplying by the price.
2. Subtract the decrease in price from the original price to find the new price.

Example: 6% decrease in cost of an object which originally cost $8.95

$6\% = 0.06$ Use the decimal equivalent

6% of 8.95 is

$0.06 \cdot 8.95 =$

$8.95	Original cost	$8.95	Original price
$\times 0.06$	Amount of decrease	-0.54	Price decrease
$0.537 = $0.54		$8.41	Total new price

Practice Set VII – 9

Find the new cost for each of the following.

1. 6.6% increase on an original price of $5.47

2. 5% decrease on an original price of $10.

3. 2% decrease from an original price of $5.39

4. 8% increase from an original price of $3.35

5. 11% increase on an original price of $6.98

Practice Set VII – 10

Evaluate each of the following. Round answer to 2 places, if needed.

1. 16% of 28

2. 90% of 1,000

3. 10% of 1,600

4. 17% of 32

5. $11\,\frac{1}{2}$% of 980

6. 13% of 78

7. $\frac{1}{4}$% of 13

8. $7\,\frac{1}{4}$% of 100

9. The waiting area is to be enlarged by 25%. The present size is 1,230 square feet.

    a. How much additional space will be available?

    b. What will be the total area when complete?

Practice Set VII – 11

The following items are taken from two price lists. Company A gives a 22% discount, while Company B's prices have increased by 7 $^{1}/_{2}$%. Find the new prices of each company.

Item	Company A list price	Company A new price	Company B list price	Company B new price
General operating scissors	$6.10		$4.45	
Metzenbaum scissors	$8.30		$6.25	
Iris scissors	$7.05		$5.00	
Allis tissue forceps	$7.58		$5.55	
Surgical cotton wadding	$4.20		$3.85	
Kelly forceps	$5.20		$3.52	
Needle holders	$4.25		$3.00	
Gauze sponges	$60.00/cs		$42.75/cs	
Endotracheal tubes	$2.38		$1.93	
First-aid dressing	$15/dz.		$14.50/dz.	
Mayo intestinal needles	$9.20/dz.		$8.75/dz.	

Solutions – General

The term *grams per deciliter* is used in hospital medicine. For example, determining the amount of hemoglobin in the blood is expressed as g/dl, which means the number of grams per 100 ml or grams per deciliter. *Gram percent* (g%) means grams per 100 ml. Both grams percent for grams per 100 ml and grams per deciliter are terms used. However, the term gram per deciliter has become popular in recent times.

Example: 12 grams in 100 ml. of solution is termed 12 gram percent or 12 g% or 12 g/dl.

Note that 100 ml = 1 deciliter $\qquad \dfrac{12\ g}{100\ ml} = \dfrac{12\ g}{1\ dl}$

Practice Set VII – 12

Express each of the following as grams per deciliter.

1. 14 g/100 ml =

2. 0.9 g/100 ml =

3. 0.5 g/100 ml =

4. 1 g/100 ml =

5. 4 g/100 ml =

Sometimes the quantity is very small and the term milligram percent (mg%) is used. This means the number of mg per 100 ml or the number of mg per deciliter.

Example: 5 mg in 100 ml of solution is termed 5 mg percent or 5 mg%

Convert:

    6. 3.2 mg/100 ml =   **7.** 0.4 mg/100 ml =

Solutions whose concentration are given in % means the number of grams (g) of a substance per 100 milliliters (ml) of solution or, if liquid, the number of milliliters of a substance per 100 milliliters of the solution. Calculate the concentration in % for each of the following.

Examples: *(i)* 12.5 g of sodium chloride in 100 ml of solution would be a 12.5% solution of sodium chloride. *(ii)* 22 ml of Formalin (a liquid chemical) in 100 ml of solution would be a 22% solution of Formalin.

    8.   0.9 g of sodium chloride in 100 ml of solution

    9.   5 g of dextrose in 100 ml of solution

    10.   4.5 g of dextrose in 100 ml of solution

    11.   10 ml of formalin in 100 ml of solution

    12.   2 g of copper sulfate in 100 ml of solution

    13.   70 ml of isopropyl alcohol in 100 ml of solution

    14.   2 ml of formalin in 100 ml of solution

Chapter 8
Ratio and Proportion

The study of ratios provides the background necessary to solve dosage problems involving ratio and proportion.

The comparison of one quantity with another like quantity is called a ratio. For example, suppose you compare a dime and a nickel. Both involve money, but are of different size and weight (among other differences.) We could compare their values and write a ratio as 10 cents to 5 cents. We could indicate this ratio as 10 : 5 using a colon to represent the ratio 10 to 5. Another way this ratio could be represented is as a fraction: $\dfrac{10}{5}$.

All the rules governing fractions apply to ratios as well.

Example:

Compare these two circles:

 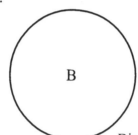

Diameter: 9

Diameter: 15

The diameter of circle A compared to the diameter of circle B may be written as the *ratio*:

$$9 \text{ to } 15 \quad \text{or} \quad 9:15 \quad \text{or} \quad \frac{9}{15}$$

This last can be reduced: $\dfrac{9}{15} = \dfrac{3}{5}$ $\quad \dfrac{3}{5}$ or $3:5$

Ratios are always expressed in lowest terms (as are fractions).

Examples: (i) 5:10 or $\dfrac{5}{10} = \dfrac{1}{2}$ or $1:2$

(ii) 3:9 or $\dfrac{3}{9} = \dfrac{1}{3}$ or $1:3$

Practice Set VIII – 1

   Read the following problems and express the information given as a ratio.

   1. If graduated cylinder "A" has 80 milliliters of solution and a second graduated cylinder "B" has 40 milliliters of the solution, what is the ratio of "A" to "B"?   [80:40 = 2:1]

   2. Refer to the previous problem (a). What is the ratio of "B" to "A"?

   3. Two young boys, "A" and "B" are weighed separately. "A" weighs 60 pounds and "B" weighs 25 pounds. What is the (weight) ratio of "A" to "B"?

   4. a. A solution mixture has the ratio of one part hydrochloric acid (HCL), 70 parts Ethyl Alcohol (EtOH), and 29 parts water. What is the ratio of EtOH to water?

   b. In part **a** of this problem, what is the ratio of water to HCL?

   The *value* of a ratio is found by dividing the numerator by the denominator to make a decimal number.

   Examples: *value*

   (i) 4:5   or $\dfrac{4}{5}$ $\longrightarrow$ $\dfrac{4}{5} = 0.8$

   (ii) 3:6   or $\dfrac{3}{6}$ $\longrightarrow$ $\dfrac{3}{6} = \dfrac{1}{2} = 0.5$

Examples: (i) 4 : 32 $\quad \dfrac{4}{32} = \dfrac{1}{8} = 0.125$

(ii) 6 : 18 $\quad ^6/_{18} = ^1/_3 = 0.33$ $\quad$ [Note the value of 6:18 is equal to the value of 1:3]

Practice Set VIII – 2

Convert each ratio to fraction form (reduce where necessary) and find the value of the ratio to nearest hundredth.

1. 5 : 15 $\qquad$ **2.** 9 : 81 $\qquad$ **3.** 17 : 51

4. 6 : 12 $\qquad$ **5.** 8 : 64 $\qquad$ **6.** 9 : 10

Ratios usually have the same units.

Examples: (i) 10 feet : 40 feet $\qquad$ (ii) 1 cc : 50 cc $\qquad$ (iii) 4 in : 40 in

However, in clinical laboratory conditions, ratios *may* have dissimilar units. Ratios with dissimilar units are called *rates*. We can reduce ratios without affecting the units.

Examples: (i) 5 mg : 1 cc $\qquad$ (ii) 1 cc : 5 lb. body wt.

$$\dfrac{5\ mg}{1\ cc} \qquad\qquad \dfrac{1\ cc}{5\ lbs}$$

$$(iii)\ 15\ g : 100\ ml = \dfrac{15\ g}{100\ ml} = \dfrac{3\ g}{20\ ml}$$

Practice Set VIII – 3

Write the ratios for the following. Be sure to include units.

1. There are 5 grams of sodium chloride found in 100 ml of a saline solution.

2. 10 mg of sodium caparsolate are dissolved in 1 ml of solution.

3. There are 100 mg of Thiamin in every 1 cc of solution.

4. The dosage for Vitamin B complex is 1 cc for every 100 lbs. body weight.

5. Thorazine contains 25 mg in every ml in liquid form.

6. 0.1 mg of Thorazine is given for every 2.0 kg of body weight.

7. 1 cc of sodium pentobarbital is given for every 5 lb of body weight.

Medicine Bottles and Labels

Working in a clinic or lab may involve using the information from a medicine bottle label or package insert to determine dosage. It is your responsibility to determine the correct dosage for the patient even if the unit dosage is provided.

A lot of information is provided on the medicine bottle label itself and / or the package insert. Your understanding and comprehension of dosage and concentration and their meanings cannot be minimized.

You may be given the opportunity to learn and practice reading and interpreting the dosage and concentration information commonly found on a label.

Dosage is the rate of administration, generally provided in terms of how much to administer per pound, kilogram, or individual body type.

Examples: 5 mg per 10 lbs or $\dfrac{5\,mg}{10\,lbs}$

1 cc per 5 lbs body weight or $\dfrac{1\,cc}{5\,lbs}$

1 capsule per individual

1 cc per 1 kg or $\dfrac{1\,cc}{1\,kg}$

Concentration is expressed in terms of how much active ingredient per unit of medication.

Examples: $\dfrac{5\,mg}{\text{tablet}}$ $\dfrac{250\,mg}{\text{capsule}}$ $\dfrac{1000\,mg}{1\,cc}$

Most dosage problems can be solved using proportions. A *proportion* is composed of two ratios that are equal. The ratios 1 : 2 and 12 : 24 form a proportion since the two ratios are equal. A proportion can be written 1 : 2 = 12 : 24 which is read " 1 is to 2 as 12 is to 24." A proportion is more commonly written as $\frac{1}{2} = \frac{12}{24}$. Typically, three of the values are known and there is an unknown fourth value. You can determine the unknown value by using a technique called cross–multiplication to solve the proportion.

The parts of a proportion: If we had two ratios such as 1 : 3 and 4 : 12 which represent equal quantities, one way they can be expressed as a proportion is …

$$1 : 3 = 4 : 12$$

extremes

means

The two outside terms of a proportion (1 and 12) are called extremes. The two inner terms (3 and 4) are called means. In any proportion, the product of the extremes equals the product of the means. $1 \times 12 = 3 \times 4$

The most common method to express a proportion is in fraction form.

Example: 1 : 3 = 4 : 12   can be written $\frac{1}{3} = \frac{4}{12}$

When written in this manner, a missing, or unknown, element of the proportion can be determined by cross-multiplying.

Example: 2 : 5 = 8 : n   or $\frac{2}{5} = \frac{8}{n}$ n represents the unknown term

cross-multiply: 2 x n = 2n   and 5 x 8 = 40

yields the equation: 2n = 40

In order to solve this equation, the 2 must be eliminated from the left–hand side of the equation. Since 2n indicates multiplication, undo that by using division. Divide each side of the equation by 2.

$$\frac{\cancel{2}n}{\cancel{2}} = \frac{40}{2}$$

dividing both sides of the equation by 2 and canceling the twos on the left-hand side

$$n = 20$$

Check for the correct solution by multiplying the means and the extremes: $2 \times 20 = 5 \times 8$!

Some helpful rules governing proportions:

Both sides of the proportion equality can be:

- multiplied by the same number without changing the value of the proportion.
- divided by the same number without changing the value of the proportion.
- added to by the same number without changing the value of the proportion.
- subtracted to or from by the same number without changing its value.
- inverted without changing its value.

Tip: to solve a proportion by cross-multiplication, multiply the two numbers diagonally opposite each other and divide by the number that is diagonally opposite the unknown.

Examples: *(i)*

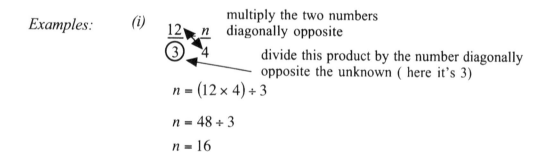

$$n = (12 \times 4) \div 3$$

$$n = 48 \div 3$$

$$n = 16$$

(ii) $\dfrac{n}{7} \diagup \dfrac{10}{35}$ multiply diagonally across the equals sign; divide by the 35 since 35 has no number to multiply by

$n = \dfrac{7 \times 10}{35}$

$n = 2$

(iii) $\dfrac{5}{n} = \dfrac{35}{56}$

$n = \dfrac{5 \times 56}{35}$

$n = 8$

Note that cancellation techniques **cannot** be used across equals signs.

Practice Set VIII – 4

Find the value of the unknown term in each of the following proportions. Round to nearest hundredth.

1. $n : 200 = 1 : 10$

2. $1 : 15 = 0.2 : n$

3. $1 : 15 = 0.1 : x$

(Notice the complex fraction in #5.)

4. $\dfrac{x}{2000} = \dfrac{.85}{100}$

5. $\dfrac{\frac{1}{6}}{\frac{1}{8}} = \dfrac{x}{30}$

6. $\dfrac{3}{6} = \dfrac{1}{x}$

7. $\dfrac{1}{5000} = \dfrac{.2}{a}$

8. $\dfrac{2}{n} = \dfrac{22}{33}$

9. $\dfrac{0.9}{100} = \dfrac{x}{1000}$

10. $\dfrac{14}{n} = \dfrac{7}{28}$

11. $\dfrac{10}{100} = \dfrac{x}{4}$

12. $\dfrac{x}{16} = \dfrac{8}{64}$

13. $5:100 = 20:x$ **14.** $\dfrac{14}{12} = \dfrac{7}{x}$ **15.** $\dfrac{1}{50} = \dfrac{x}{\frac{1}{2}}$

16. If 9 medicine carts cost $450, how many carts can be purchased for $1000 ?

17. If 8 hemostats cost $72, how much will 19 hemostats cost?

18. The number of WBC (white blood cells) can be estimated using viscosity measurements. Assuming a linear relationship, what is the estimated WBC count when the average flow time is 5 seconds if a 5000 WBC has an average flow time of 6 seconds?

Problems found in a clinical setting usually have units associated with them. When solving these problems, make certain to include the units. Units, by the way, will "cancel" just as numbers do when multiplying and dividing fractions.

Note: since the letter "*x*" is frequently used to signify, or stand in for, an unknown quantity, we will use the more conventional "dot (•) or an asterisk (*)" to signify multiplication.

Example: $\dfrac{x}{5\ lbs} = \dfrac{2\ mg}{10\ lbs}$ cross-multiply as usual

$x = \dfrac{2\ mg \cdot 5\ \cancel{lbs}}{10\ \cancel{lbs}}$ the pounds units cancel

$x = \dfrac{2\ mg \cdot \cancel{5}^{\,1}}{\cancel{10}_{\,2}}$ cancel numbers if possible

$x = \dfrac{\cancel{2}\ mg}{\cancel{2}}$ continue canceling; remember $\dfrac{2}{2} = 1$

$x = 1\ mg$

The units can also be used to check the result. If the answer had been in pounds, there would have been some type of error somewhere. A useful procedure is to make sure the units in the two numerators match each other and the units in the two denominators also match one another.

Practice Set VIII – 5

Solve the following proportions. Be sure your answer includes the proper units.

1. $\dfrac{300\ mg}{x} = \dfrac{10\ mg}{1\ ml}$

2. $\dfrac{2\ lbs}{4\ cc} = \dfrac{10\ lbs}{x}$

3. $\dfrac{x}{10\ lbs} = \dfrac{1\ cc}{25\ lbs}$

4. $\dfrac{x}{1400\ lbs} = \dfrac{5\ mg}{100\ lbs}$

Chapter 8 Review

Solve each of the following. Be sure to show units where applicable. Round answers to 3 decimal places when necessary.

1. $\dfrac{x}{2} = \dfrac{3}{6}$

2. $\dfrac{x}{8} = \dfrac{10}{16}$

3. $\dfrac{x}{17} = \dfrac{3}{51}$

4. $\dfrac{x}{9} = \dfrac{21}{24}$

5. $\dfrac{x}{6} = \dfrac{3}{16}$

6. $\dfrac{x}{7} = \dfrac{5}{9}$

7. $\dfrac{x}{3} = \dfrac{9}{1}$

8. $\dfrac{x}{2.5} = \dfrac{8}{3}$

9. $\dfrac{8}{x} = \dfrac{16}{3}$

10. $\dfrac{4}{x} = \dfrac{7}{11}$

11. $\dfrac{3}{4} = \dfrac{75}{x}$

12. $\dfrac{2.5}{6} = \dfrac{x}{25}$

13. $\dfrac{13}{14} = \dfrac{10}{x}$

14. $\dfrac{12}{30} = \dfrac{x}{5}$

15. $\dfrac{13}{39} = \dfrac{9}{x}$

16. $\dfrac{14}{28} = \dfrac{x}{8.5}$

17. $\dfrac{3}{9} = \dfrac{5}{x}$

18. $\dfrac{1.8\ mg}{1\ cc} = \dfrac{3.5\ mg}{x}$

19. $\dfrac{1\ cc}{5\ lbs} = \dfrac{x}{35\ lbs}$

20. $\dfrac{1\ cc}{10\ lbs} = \dfrac{x}{35\ lbs}$

21. $\dfrac{1\ cc}{5\ lbs} = \dfrac{x}{65\ lbs}$

22. $\dfrac{x}{7.5\ lbs} = \dfrac{0.25\ mg}{1\ lb}$

23. $\dfrac{1\ drop}{5\ cc} = \dfrac{n}{35\ cc}$

24. $\dfrac{10\ mg}{1\ ml} = \dfrac{70\ mg}{x}$

25. $\dfrac{55\ mg}{n} = \dfrac{10\ mg}{1\ ml}$

26. $\dfrac{0.5\ mg}{1\ cc} = \dfrac{7.5\ mg}{a}$

27. $\dfrac{1\ cc}{25\ lbs} = \dfrac{a}{58\ lbs}$

28. $\dfrac{x}{500 \; ml} = \dfrac{4 \; g}{100 \; ml}$

29. $\dfrac{a}{1000 \; ml} = \dfrac{0.9 \; g}{100 \; ml}$

30. $\dfrac{160 \; mg}{n} = \dfrac{40 \; mg}{1 \; cc}$

31. $\dfrac{x}{17 \; lbs} = \dfrac{1 \; mg}{1 \; lb}$

32. $\dfrac{x}{30 \; cc} = \dfrac{1 \; drop}{5 \; cc}$

33. $\dfrac{x}{5.5 \; lbs} = \dfrac{0.5 \; mg}{1 \; lb}$

34. $\dfrac{x}{5.5 \; lbs} = \dfrac{0.25 \; mg}{1 \; lb}$

35. $\dfrac{x}{800 \; ml} = \dfrac{2.5 \; g}{100 \; ml}$

36. $\dfrac{160 \; mg}{x} = \dfrac{20 \; mg}{1 \; cc}$

37. $\dfrac{180 \; mg}{x} = \dfrac{6 \; mg}{10 \; cc}$

38. $\dfrac{x}{25 \; lbs} = \dfrac{\frac{1}{4} \; mg}{1 \; lb}$

39. $\dfrac{x}{24 \; cc} = \dfrac{1 \; drop}{5 \; cc}$

40. $\dfrac{325 \; mg}{x} = \dfrac{25 \; mg}{1 \; ml}$

41. $\dfrac{x}{14 \; lb} = \dfrac{0.25 \; mg}{1 \; lb}$

42. $\dfrac{20 \; mg}{1 \; cc} = \dfrac{3.50 \; mg}{x}$

43. $\dfrac{x}{1600\ lbs} = \dfrac{2\ mg}{100\ lbs}$

44. $\dfrac{32\ mg}{x} = \dfrac{10\ mg}{1\ ml}$

45. $\dfrac{x}{1250\ lbs} = \dfrac{4\ mg}{100\ lbs}$

46. $\dfrac{x}{2000\ lbs} = \dfrac{3\ mg}{100\ lbs}$

47. $\dfrac{n}{25\ lbs} = \dfrac{1\ cc}{5\ lbs}$

48. $\dfrac{5\ mg}{n} = \dfrac{6\ mg}{1\ ml}$

49. $\dfrac{13\ mg}{x} = \dfrac{25\ mg}{1\ ml}$

50. $\dfrac{n}{7.5\ lbs} = \dfrac{0.1\ mg}{1\ lb}$

51. $\dfrac{18\ mg}{x} = \dfrac{20\ mg}{1\ ml}$

52. $\dfrac{0.5\ mg}{1\ lb} = \dfrac{x}{8.5\ lbs}$

53. $\dfrac{x}{9\ lbs} = \dfrac{1\ cc}{25\ lbs}$

54. $\dfrac{x}{13\ lbs} = \dfrac{\frac{1}{4}\ mg}{1\ lb}$

55. $\dfrac{n}{21\ lbs} = \dfrac{1\ cc}{5\ lbs}$

56. $\dfrac{23\ mg}{x} = \dfrac{40\ mg}{1\ cc}$

57. $\dfrac{2.4\ mg}{x} = \dfrac{6\ mg}{1\ ml}$

Chapter 9
Measurement Systems

Technicians need to be familiar with a variety of laboratory equipment – graduated cylinders of various sizes, syringes and different types of tips and needles, eyedroppers and other glassware used for preparing, mixing and dispensing medicines and chemicals used in the practice of medicine. Measuring devices come in a variety of shapes and sizes. It is important to pick an appropriately sized container and measure accurately.

Reading and recording results from measurements are equally important. Great care must be taken when reading graduated cylinders and measuring devices such as spectrometers. The technician should read a device at eye level. Do not raise the item to your level, rather place the item on a flat surface and get down to look at it directly.

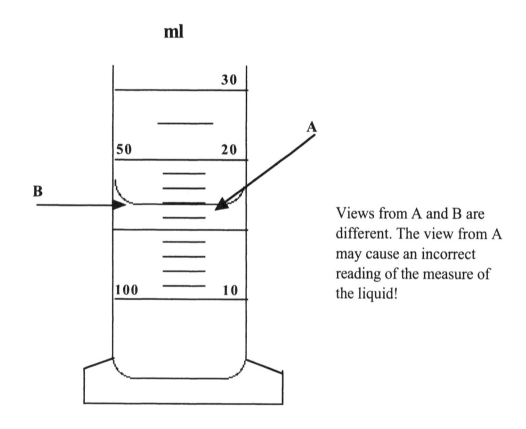

Views from A and B are different. The view from A may cause an incorrect reading of the measure of the liquid!

Common errors that occur when measuring chemicals or medicines include the phenomena of parallax. *Parallax* is the apparent displacement of an object when viewed from two different points.

ml

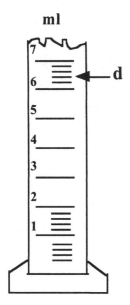

Measurements must also take into account the scale of the container. In this case, the numbers are in milliliters and the marks indicate an increase by "twos" from milliliter to milliliter. Shown (d) is the measure for 6.4 ml.

Capillary action occurs when liquid wets the container it is in and causes a rise along the contact surface. The portion of the liquid not in contact with the surface does not rise. This capillary action can be seen in a graduated cylinder. The result is a curved upper surface of a liquid column called the meniscus. The *meniscus* is the concave, or curved up at the edge, surface of the liquid measurement. The correct reading is taken along the bottom of the depression.

Capillary action can also be seen if a fine bore tube is inserted into a container of liquid, the level of liquid in the tube will be higher than its level in the surrounding liquid in the container. The finer the bore of the tube, the higher the liquid will be drawn up the tube.

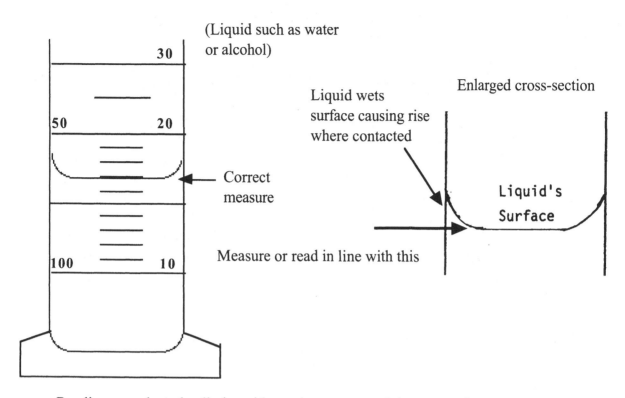

Meniscus

(Liquid such as water or alcohol)

Reading a graduated cylinder with meniscus can result in an error in measurement. Always read straight across the cylinder, lining up the marked measurements along the outside of the cylinder with the bottom of the meniscus.

An error can occur when reading instrument scales. If a scale is viewed off-center, the reading may be incorrect. Most instruments have a reflective strip that allows the reader to hide the reflection of the needle directly behind the needle itself, thus assuring you are correctly reading the instrument.

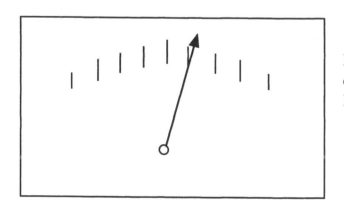

Read instrument scales carefully. Read directly from the front and at the same level as the instrument.

The technician should be equally aware of common terms likely to be encountered in a clinic or lab such as density and specific gravity.

Density is defined as the amount of mass (or weight) per unit volume. For example,

$$\frac{grams}{milliliter} \qquad\qquad \frac{kilogram}{liter} \qquad\qquad \frac{lbs}{foot^3}$$

abbreviations can include: g/ml, g/cc, kg/L, lb/ft3

The density of lead is greater than the density of water which indicates that the mass per unit volume of lead is greater than the mass per unit of volume of water.

Specific gravity is a means of comparing densities to that of water. Note that specific gravity is a number with no units.

$$\text{Specific gravity} = \frac{\text{Density of a substance}}{\text{Density of water}}$$

Examples: Density of Lead: 11.3 g / cc   and density of urine 1.025 g / cc

Then …

(i) Specific gravity of Lead $= \dfrac{11.3 \text{ g / cc}}{1 \text{ g / cc}} = 11.3$

(ii) Specific gravity of urine $= \dfrac{1.025 \text{ g / cc}}{1 \text{ g / cc}} = 1.025$

Practice Set IX – 1

1.  This curved surface of the liquid is called a _____

2. Water can be pulled up a fine bored tube by _____

3. The density of water is _____ g / cc.

4. The density of gold is 19.3 g / cc, determine its specific gravity.

5. The density of silver is 10.5 g / cc. Find the specific gravity of silver.

The Metric System

The metric system of measurement is the most widely used system in the world. It is a measurement system based upon powers of ten. The basic units of measurement are the meter for length, the liter for volume, and the gram for mass (weight). Multiples and fractional parts are formed by adding a prefix to the basic unit. The prefixes most commonly used are presented here.

Decimal System	Numerical meaning	Metric Prefix	Abbreviation
Million	1,000,000	Mega-	M
Thousand	1,000	kilo-	k
Hundred	100	hecto-	h
Ten	10	deka-	da
Unit	1	None	None
Tenth	0.1	deci-	d
Hundredth	0.01	centi-	c
Thousandth	0.001	milli-	m
Millionth	0.000001	micro-	mc or μ
Billionth	0.000000001	nano-	n
Trillionth	1×10^{-12}	pico-	p

Practice Set IX – 2

Write the appropriate metric prefix:

1. Hundreds   _____

2. Tenths   _____

3. Units   _____

4. Thousands   _____

5. Thousandths   _____

6. Tens   _____

7. Hundredths   _____

Common abbreviations along with the words for mass, length and volume are given in the chart below. A special note: the abbreviation for deka- has changed several times over the years. The student should be aware that s/he may encounter such variations as decameter (dam), decagram (dag) and decaliter (dal). We will use deka– (dk) , unless otherwise noted.

Prefix	Length	Weight	Volume
kilo-	kilometer (km)	kilogram (kg)	kiloliter (kl)
hecto-	hectometer (hm)	hectogram (hg)	hectoliter (hl)
deka-	dekameter (dkm)	dekagram (dkg)	dekaliter (dkl)
basic unit	meter (m)	gram (g)	liter (l)
deci-	decimeter (dm)	decigram (dg)	deciliter (dl)
centi-	centimeter (cm)	centigram (cg)	centiliter (cl)
milli-	millimeter (mm)	milligram (mg)	milliliter (ml)
micro-	micrometer (μm)	microgram (μg)	microliter (μl)

The ability to recreate the following chart will prove to be an invaluable aid in mastering the metric system and for making conversions within this system.

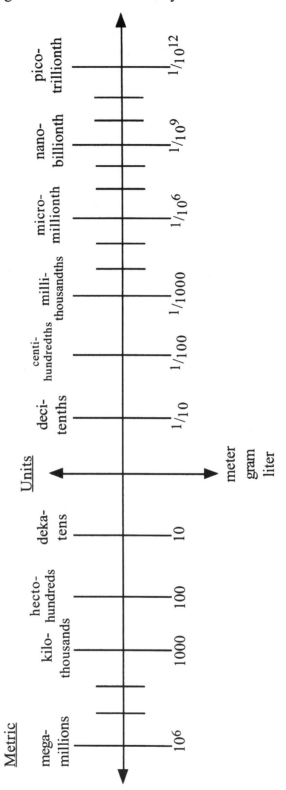

Metric				Units									
mega- millions		kilo- thousands	hecto- hundreds	deka- tens		meter gram liter	deci- tenths	centi- hundredths	milli- thousandths	micro- millionth	nano- billionth		pico- trillionth
10^6		1000	100	10			$1/10$	$1/100$	$1/1000$	$1/10^6$	$1/10^9$		$1/10^{12}$

Practice Set IX – 3

Write the abbreviation and the value of the number of units for each of the following.

Metric Units	Abbreviation	Value
kilometer	**km**	**1000 meters**
1. decimeter	_____	_____
2. milligram	_____	_____
3. dekagram	_____	_____
4. meter	_____	_____
5. deciliter	_____	_____
6. dekameter	_____	_____
7. gram	_____	_____
8. hectometer	_____	_____
9. decigram	_____	_____
10. centiliter	_____	_____
11. liter	_____	_____
12. dekaliter	_____	_____
13. hectoliter	_____	_____
14. kiloliter	_____	_____
15. milliliter	_____	_____
16. centimeter	_____	_____

Conversion from one metric unit to another

Conversion from one unit to another involves merely moving the decimal point the same number of "steps" in the same direction as it takes to get from one unit to the other.

Examples: (i) 8 km = _?_ cm

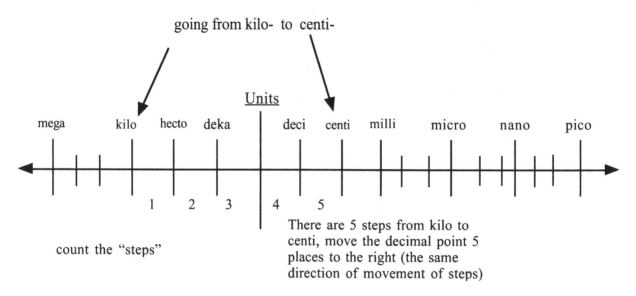

going from kilo- to centi-

Units

mega   kilo   hecto   deka   deci   centi   milli   micro   nano   pico

                    1   2   3   4   5

count the "steps"

There are 5 steps from kilo to centi, move the decimal point 5 places to the right (the same direction of movement of steps)

Thus, 8 km = 800000 cm

(ii) 4000.2 mg = ? kg

That's six steps to the left. Move the decimal point the same 6 places to left.

4000.2 mg = ? kg

move 6 places in this direction

Result? 0.0040002 kg

Note: Between milli- and micro-, micro- and nano-, nano- and pico-, mega- and kilo- , there are two unnamed units that must each be considered (counted) as steps.

Practice Set IX – 4

Convert from one unit to another for each of the following.

1.   0.12 km = _____ dm

2.   12.0 g   = _____ mg

3.   0.21 hl = _____ cl

4.   1.5 cm = _____ mm

5.   5.51 dkg = _____ cg

6.   0.6125 hg = _____ mg

7.   3.0 kl   = _____ L

8.   401.0 L = _____ cl

9.   515.12 dkl = _____ ml

10.   12.14 km = _____ m

11.   11.2 mg = _____ dg

12.   2.1 dl   = _____ kl

13.   12.3 mm = _____ m

14.   51 g   = _____ kg

15.   23.5 cm = _____ dkm

16.   65.3 L = _____ hl

17.   3.4 m = _____ km

18.   63.5 dm = _____ dkm

19.   151123.5 ml = _____ kl

Apothecary and English Measurement Systems
Inter– and Intra–System Conversions

Medicines, and other materials, are sometimes measured using an antiquated system called the Apothecaries' system. It is essential for medical personnel to be as familiar with this system as with the metric and English systems since each of these systems of measurement are likely to be encountered in the laboratory, office, or clinic.

The following are common units and abbreviations of length, volume, and weight in English and apothecary systems of measurements.

Length	Volume	Weight
Inches – in	Fluid Ounces – fl. oz.	Grains – gr
Feet – ft	Pints – pts	Ounces – oz
Yards – yds	Quarts – qts	Pounds – lbs
Miles – mi	Gallons – gal	Tons – T

There are also common household measurements with which you should be familiar.

Cups – c   Tablespoons – Tbs or Tbsp or T   Teaspoons – tsp; or t

Equivalents

Length

12 in = 1 ft

36 in = 1 yd

3 ft = 1 yd

5,280 ft = 1 mi

Volume

16 oz = 1 pt

32 fl oz = 1 qt

2 pt = 1 qt

4 qt = 1 gal

8 pt = 1 gal

128 fl oz = 1 gal

1 pt = 2 cups

1 qt = 4 cups

2 Tbs = 1 fl oz

3 tsp = 1 Tbs

6 tsp = 1 fl oz

1 cup = 8 fl oz

Weight

16 oz = 1 lb

2000 lb = 1 ton

Temperature Conversions

$$C = \frac{5}{9}\left(F - 32\right)$$

or

$$C = \left(F - 32\right) \div 1.8$$

$$F = \frac{9}{5}C + 32$$

or

$$F = 1.8C + 32$$

Approximate Equivalents Between Systems

1 g = 15 gr

65 mg = 1 gr

30 g = 1 oz

454 g = 1 lb

1 kg = 2.2 lb

1 oz = 438 gr

1 cup = 237 ml

1 fl oz = 30 ml

1 tsp = 5 cc

1 pt = 473 ml

1 qt = 946 ml

1 gal = 3.785 L

1 in = 2.5 cm

1 m = 39.4 in

1 m = 1.09 yd

1 Tbs = 15 ml

Practice Set IX – 5

Write the abbreviation or the name for each of the following.

1. pint _____

2. T _____

3. cup _____

4. lb _____

5. t _____

6. mile _____

7. oz _____

8. fluid ounce _____

9. ounces _____

10. yard _____

11. gallon _____

12. qt _____

13. inch _____

14. feet _____

15. grains _____

Sometimes it is necessary to convert from one unit to another within a system. Unlike the metric system, this conversion can be more difficult and laborious. Since it is not based on unit of ten, the decimal point cannot be moved to obtain the answer. One must use ratio and proportion, conversion factors to convert units, or dimensional analysis.

Example: Convert 2.5 gal into qt

$$1 \text{ gal} = 4 \text{ qt}$$

ratio / proportion

$$\frac{x \ qt}{2.5 \ gal} = \frac{4 \ qt}{1 \ gal}$$

$$x \ qt = \frac{4 \ qt \times 2.5 \ gal}{1 \ gal}$$

$$x = 10 \ qt$$

conversion

conversion factor: $\dfrac{4 \ qt}{1 \ gal}$

$$x = 2.5 \ gal \left(\frac{4 \ qt}{1 \ gal} \right)$$

$$x = 10 \ qt$$

Examples (dimensional analysis):

(i) Convert 7 pts to cups. 2 cups = 1 pt

$$\frac{7 \text{ pints}}{} \bigg| \frac{2 \text{ cups}}{1 \text{ pint}} = 14 \text{ cups}$$ 7 pints is equal to 14 cups

(ii) Convert 2.5 gals to fluid ounces. 128 fl oz = 1 gal

$$\frac{2.5 \text{ gal}}{} \bigg| \frac{128 \text{ fl oz}}{1 \text{ gal}} = 320 \text{ fl oz}$$

(iii) Convert 2.5 days into minutes. 1 day = 24 hrs, 1 hr = 60 min

$$\frac{2.5 \text{ days}}{} \bigg| \frac{24 \text{ hr}}{1 \text{ day}} \bigg| \frac{60 \text{ min}}{1 \text{ hr}} = 3600 \text{ min}$$

Practice Set IX – 6

Convert the following into the desired units. Use any method.

1. 2.5 gal = _____ qts

2. 256 fl oz = _____ gal

3. 6 T = _____ t

4. 27 fl oz = _____ T

5. 5 pts = _____ c

6. 2.5 lbs. = _____ oz

7. $2\frac{1}{4}$ ft = _____ in

8. $4\frac{1}{3}$ yd = _____ ft

9. 18 fl oz = _____ tsp

10. 14 ft = _____ in

11. 3 oz = _____ gr.

12. 1.5 qt = _____ fl oz

13. 2 mi = _____ ft

14. 1.7 tons = _____ lbs.

15. 3 tablespoons = _____ tsp

16. 25 oz = _____ lbs.

Practice Set IX – 7

Convert. Use any method.

1. 16 fl oz _____ pts

2. 32 fl oz _____ pts _____ qts

3. 128 fl oz _____ pts _____ qts _____ gals

4. 3 gals _____ qts _____ pts _____ fl oz

5. 16 oz _____ lbs.

6. 3 lbs. _____ oz

7. 6 ft _____ in

8. 36 ft _____ yds

9. 7 in _____ ft

10. 72 oz _____ lbs.

11. 3 Tbsp _____ fl oz

12. 1 Tbsp _____ tsp

13. 1 tsp _____ T

14. 30 fl oz _____ tsp

15. 30 fl oz _____ tablespoons

16. 8 oz _____ lbs.

17. 24 lbs. _____ oz

18. 10 Tbsp _____ tsp

It is often necessary to convert from the metric to the English or apothecaries' systems (or back). For example, if an patient is weighed in pounds and the dosage is in kilograms.

Generally, the equivalents used for everyday simple tasks are not as accurate as shown. Frequently, for example, liters and quarts are considered equivalent. For some non-critical applications this may be acceptable. However, the use of such rough apporximations is not acceptable in scientific or research work.

Examples:

(i)   Actual   Common rough approximation
        1 qt. = 946 ml   1 qt = 1000 ml = 1 L

(ii) It may be common to use the following measures for cups/milliliters

1 cup = 237 ml   and   1 pt = 500 ml   but   1 pt = 2 cups

Of course, there is no substitute for good judgment. One should not convert gallons to milliliters and then the milliliters to fluid ounces (*inter*system.)

It is easier, more efficient, and more accurate to convert directly from gallons to fluid ounces (*intra–system*).

1 gal = 128 fl oz

Still, there are occasions when you must convert from one value to another, from one system to another, or even make several conversions at a time. However, this should be done only as a last resort or when no better alternative is available. A liter and a quart, for instance, are generally considered approximately equivalent for quick conversions.

Q.   1 L = ??? tsp

A.   1 L = 1000 ml = 200 tsp

The conversion from one system to another can be done in three ways: ratios and proportions; dimensional analysis; or simple conversion factors .

Example: Convert 2.5 liters to gallons

Ratio and Proportion

$$\frac{x}{2.5L} = \frac{1gal}{3.785L}$$

$$x = \frac{2.5L \cdot 1gal}{3.785L}$$

$x = 0.66$ gal

Conversion Factor

$$x = 2.5L\left(\frac{1gal}{3.785L}\right)$$

$x = 0.66$ gal

Dimensional Analysis

$$\frac{2.5\,\cancel{L} \mid 1 \text{ gallon}}{\mid 3.785\,\cancel{L}} = 0.66 \text{ gallons}$$

The use of dimensional analysis shows it is a useful technique for keeping track of the proper units when doing a problem. Dimensional analysis is commonly used in chemistry.

Examples: (i) Change 74 pounds to kilograms

$$\frac{74 \; \cancel{lb} \; | \; 1 \; kg}{| \; 2.2 \; \cancel{lb}} \;=\; \frac{74 \; kg}{2.2} \;=\; \frac{74}{2.2} kg \;\approx\; 33.6 \; kg$$

(ii) 25 $^g/_{100 \; ml}$ rewritten in terms of milligrams is

$$\frac{25 \; \cancel{g} \; | \; \overset{10}{\cancel{1000}} \, mg}{\cancel{100} \, ml \; | \; 1 \, \cancel{g}} \;=\; 250 \; ^{mg}\!/_{ml}$$

(iii) Convert 75 grains into ounces.

$$\frac{75 \; \cancel{gr} \; | \; 1 \; oz}{| \; 438 \; \cancel{gr}} \;=\; 0.17 \; oz$$

Practice Set IX – 8

Convert. Use proportions or dimensional analysis.

1. 35 ml = _____ tsp

2. 4.5 L = _____ gal

3. 5 in = _____ cm

4. $3\frac{1}{2}$ fl oz = _____ cc

5. 2700 ml = _____ qt

6. 3 Tbs. = _____ cc

7. 45 g = _____ oz

8. 2.4 gr. = _____ mg

9. 3 g = _____ gr.

10. 27 kg = _____ lbs.

11. 2 lb = _____ g

12. 3 m = _____ in

Temperature Conversion

The two most common temperature scales are *Celsius* and *Fahrenheit*.

To convert from Fahrenheit to Celsius: $C = \frac{5}{9}(F - 32)$ or $C = (F - 32)/1.8$

To convert from Celsius to Fahrenheit: $F = \frac{9}{5}C + 32$ or $F = 1.8C + 32$

The boiling point of water is 212° F or 100° C. Each of these represents the same temperature needed to boil water. Each merely represents a different scale of measurement. The freezing point of water is 32° F or 0° C. Both describe the same condition with regards to heat (or lack of heat = cold.)

To convert from one temperature scale to another, use the given formula, substitute the known value and simplify.

Examples:

F ➤ C

70° F = ? C

$$C = \frac{5}{9}\left(70° - 32°\right)$$

$$C \approx 21.1°$$

C ➤ F

18° C = ? F

$$F = \frac{9}{5}\left(18°\right) + 32°$$

$$F = 64.4°$$

Practice Set IX – 9

Convert (round to nearest tenth degree where necessary):

1.   40° C = _____ °F

2.   60° F = _____ °C

3.   37° C = _____ °F

4.   65° F = _____ °C

5.   32° F = _____ °C

6.   70° F = _____ °C

7.   45° C = _____ °F   8.   73° F = _____ °C

9.   100° F = _____ °C   10. 78° C = _____ °F

11.   0° F = _____ °C   12. 80° C = _____ °F

13. – 10° F = _____ °C   14. 80° F = _____ °C

15. 25° C = _____ °F   16. 50° C = _____ °F

17. 10° F = _____ °C   18. 18° C = _____ °F

Practice Set IX – 10

Convert as indicated (round to hundredths if necessary):

1.   3 g = _____ gr.   2.   5 oz = _____ g

3.   130 mg = _____ gr.   4.   4.5 oz = _____ g

5.   3 oz = _____ g   6.   35 ml = _____ tsp

7. $2\frac{1}{2}$ lbs. = _____ g   **8.** 5 lb = _____ kg

9. 2.5 cups = _____ cc   **10.** 8 fl oz = _____ ml

11. 4 tsp = _____ ml   **12.** 3 pts = _____ ml

13. 7.5 pts = _____ L   **14.** 45 ml = _____ Tbs.

15. 12 in = _____ cm   **16.** 350 g = _____ lbs.

17. 45 g = _____ oz   **18.** 55 ml = _____ fl oz

19. 100 ml = _____ fl oz   **20.** 3 tsp = _____ ml

Practice Set IX – 11

Convert. Round to two places, if necessary.

1.   32 oz = _____lbs.

2.   18 pts = _____qts

3.   16 pts = _____gal

4.   6 tsp = _____Tbs.

5.   8 tsp = _____ml

6.   1 gal = _____ml

7.   5 tsp = _____Tbs.

8.   3 cups = _____ fl oz

9.   3 pts = _____cups

10.   12 cups = _____ pts

11.   100 ml = _____Tbs.

12.   1 cup = _____ fl oz

13.   5 ml = _____tsp

14.   3 oz = _____ g

15.   10 ml = _____Tbs.

16.   3 gr. = _____ mg

17.   500 ml = _____ pts   **18.**   5 g = _____ gr.

19.   1000 ml = _____ pts   **20.** $1\frac{1}{2}$ g = _____ gr.

21.   12 L = _____ qts   **22.**   7 ml = _____ tsp

23.   200 ml = _____ qts   **24.** $2\frac{1}{2}$ fl oz = _____ Tbs.

25.   6 pts = _____ qts   **26.**   150 mg = _____ gr

27.   13 qts = _____ gal   **28.**   48 g = _____ oz

29.   12 ml = _____ tsp   **30.**   85 gr. = _____ g

31.   12 ml = _____ Tbs.   **32.**   30 ml = _____ Tbs.

33.   750 ml = _____ pts   **34.**   145 g = _____ oz

35.   5 oz = _____ g   **36.**   6 qts = _____ fl oz

Practice Set IX – 12

Convert. Round to hundredths, if necessary.

1.   5 cg =_____ g

2.   1 g = _____mg

3.   2 cups = _____ pints = _____ qts = _____ cc

4.   11 pints = _____qts

5.   500 cc = _____liters

6.   2.5 L = _____ml = _____ cc

7.   0.25 L = _____ ml

8.   0.1 g = _____ mg

9.   1 fl oz = _____ ml

10.   1 qt = _____ fl oz

11.   1 g = _____ grains

12.   4 cups = _____ cc = _____ pts = _____ qts

13.   5 cc = _____ tsp

14.   1 g = _____ mg

15.   6 fl oz = _____ cc

16.   2 kg = _____ lbs.

17.   150 mg = _____ g

18.   1 gr. = _____ mg

19.   1 gal = _____ qts = _____ pts = _____ cc

20.   8 g = _____ mg

21.   0.5 g = _____ mg

22.   600 cc = _____ L

23.   250 mg = _____ g

24.   1000 mg = _____ g

25.   15 g = _____ cg

26.   11 kg = _____ lbs.

27.   1000 cc = _____ L

28.   32 fl oz = _____ qt

29.   2 g = _____ gr.

30.   4000 cc = _____ gal

31.   4 pts = _____ qts

Unit III

Chapter 10
Algebra

The study of algebra is an essential component of mathematics. Algebra involves the manipulation of symbols in order to recognize patterns and solve problems. There are few rules, but they apply to all real numbers and form the foundation of algebra. In this section, you'll learn these basic rules, how to apply the rules and use that information to solve problems.

This is not unlike what you do every day. You determine your work flow and the most efficient way to accomplish your daily tasks. You deal with problems as they arise and you interact with coworkers, supervisors and clients. We all constantly make decisions based upon the information we have to that point. As new information becomes available, we make adjustments. The study of algebra sharpens these logical and problem–solving skills.

You may have heard that learning algebra is like learning a language. Indeed, that is a good analogy. The numbers are the words and the rules and operations the grammar. In this section, the rules are presented along with the proper techniques to order the operations of arithmetic – addition, subtraction, multiplication and division. Simple equation solving follows and then practice using these tools to solve application problems. The last part of this chapter is a brief introduction to recording and reading graphs.

Rules of Real Numbers

Real number are those we use every day. They include positive and negative whole numbers (integers), fractions (rational numbers), and irrational numbers which are non–terminating, non–repeating decimals: numbers like π or $\sqrt{5}$ or $3.21435241\ldots$. Whatever the number, its use is controlled by a set of rules or properties. You probably encountered some of these rules in other classes. They include things like the commutative and associative properties. It is less important that you know the names for these rules, but it is critical that you become familiar with their uses. For it is these few simple rules which govern exactly how we use numbers – all numbers.

In no particular order, first we have the commutative and associative properties of addition and multiplication. The purpose of these rules is to control the way we add and multiply. For instance, the fact that 2 times 3 is the same as 3 times 2 means that the order in which we multiply has no bearing on the actual outcome. The answer is six either way. This property is called the commutative property and holds true for addition as well.

Examples:
$$a + b = b + a \qquad a \times b = b \times a$$
$$2 + 5 = 5 + 2 = 7 \qquad 2 \times 5 = 5 \times 2 = 10$$
$$17 + 4 = 4 + 17 = 21 \qquad 3 \times 6 = 6 \times 3 = 18$$

The associative property allows us to group the numbers in any convenient manner so that we may add and multiply in a way that is easy and fast. The associative property says that if we add, say three different numbers, it doesn't matter how we group them to perform the addition. We can add the first two and then add the third. Or we could add the second and third and then the first.

Examples:
$$(a + b) + c = a + (b + c) \qquad (a \times b) \times c = a \times (b \times c)$$
$$(5 + 2) + 3 = 5 + (2 + 3) \qquad (5 \times 2) \times 3 = 5 \times (2 \times 3)$$
$$7 + 3 = 5 + 5 \qquad 10 \times 3 = 5 \times 6$$
$$10 = 10 \qquad 30 = 30$$

By combining these properties, we can add and multiply in any fast, easy and convenient manner we like.

Examples:

(i)
$$5 + 4 + 5 + 6 = ?$$
$$5 + 5 + 4 + 6 =$$
$$(5 + 5) + (4 + 6) =$$
$$10 \ + \ 10 \ = 20$$

Using the commutative property on the 4 and 5 in the middle; then grouping the first and last pairs that were easily recognized to be 10; finally simplifying to the answer.

(ii)
$$7 \times 3 \times 8 \times 5 \times 2$$
$$(7 \times 3) \times (5 \times 2) \times 8$$
$$21 \ \times \ 10 \ \times 8$$
$$(21 \times 10) \ \times \ 8$$

Use the rules to group the numbers in any convenient manner.

Combine and simplify.

$$210$$
$$\underline{\times \ 8}$$
$$1680$$

The next couple of rules have to do with identity or unity. Their effect is to keep the basic value of a number the same. For example, if we add zero to any number the number value stays the same. Likewise, any number multiplied by a value of 1 stays the same.

Examples:

$$7 + 0 = 7 \qquad\qquad 8 \times 1 = 8$$
$$12 + 0 = 12 \qquad\qquad 11 \times 1 = 11$$
$$-3 + 0 = -3 \qquad\qquad -5 \times 1 = -5$$

Hence, the additive identity is zero. The multiplicative identity is one.

Now, here's a little reason that matters. The inverse property, when applied to a number, yields the identity! The additive inverse of a number is its opposite: -3 is the opposite of 3. -3 and 3 are additive inverses. 7 is the opposite of -7 and, thus, its additive inverse. $\dfrac{1}{4}$ is the multiplicative inverse of 4. The multiplicative inverse of a number is its reciprocal. $2/3$ is the reciprocal of $3/2$ and, therefore, its multiplicative inverse.

Examples:
$$4 + (-4) = 0 \qquad \frac{1}{3} \times 3 = 1$$
$$5 + (-5) = 0$$
$$-8 + 8 = 0 \qquad 5 \times \frac{1}{5} = 1$$

The inverse and identity properties helped you to determine common denominators and reduce fractions. These properties will be useful for solving equations as well.

The distributive property works just like it sounds. A number being multiplied to a group gets distributed, or "doled out" to each member.

Examples:
$$3 \times (2 + 4 + 5)$$
$$(3 \times 2) + (3 \times 4) + (3 \times 5)$$
$$6 + 12 + 15$$
$$(6 + 15) + 12$$
$$21 + 12 = 33$$

The 3 is distributed to every member in the numbers grouped by the parenthesis. Then the multiplication is carried out and finally the results are summed. It can be convenient to use associative and commutative properties to simplify.

(ii)
$$(2 + 3) \times 7 = 5 \times 7 = 35$$

You can see that we get the same answer using the distributive property.

$$(2 \times 7) + (3 \times 7) = 14 + 21 = 35$$

Order of Operations

You may remember the order of operations as having something to do with Aunt Sally. Unfortunately, many students mistakenly remember the actual rules the mnemonic suggests. For instance, the problem $6 \times 2 \div 3 \times 4 = ?$. Many students believe the answer to be one. This is incorrect. The correct answer is 16!

Students think of the Aunt Sally mnemonic and conclude that multiplication occurs before division. Not true! The true order of operations has multiplication and division performed from left to right throughout the problem. So the exercise becomes 6 times 2 divided by 3 times 4. Or 16.

We believe it is more helpful to learn the correct order of operations, which occur within four steps:

1. Parenthesis and other grouping symbols (brackets, braces, a fraction bar) – perform all arithmetic within parenthesis first. If there are multiple sets of grouping symbols within one another, work "inside out".

2. Powers and roots should come next. Raise any numbers to the required power and/or determine any square roots (or any other root.)

3. Perform multiplication and division, *in order*, from left to right.

4. Perform any addition and subtraction, *in order*, from left to right.

Terminology

A *variable* is a letter that can simply be a placeholder, or a representative for a number that changes. For example, in the equation $x + 2 = 5$, the letter x is a variable that holds the place for the solution of 3. In the expression $3x + 1$, the letter x can be replaced with any number and the value of the expression will change depending upon how that number varies. The examples shown include the numbers 2, 5, and 1 – all of which are *constants*.

Equations have equals signs, *expressions* do not. We solve equations and simplify expressions. If there are no equal signs in the problem, do not attempt to come up with some solution like $x = 4$. It is not possible to "solve" an expression.

Evaluate means to tell the value of an expression or an equation by making any substitutions and performing the order of operations to simplify.

Exponents...

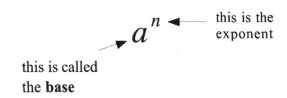

this is called the **base** a^n this is the exponent

For any real number(s):

(i) $a^n = a \cdot a \cdot a \cdot a \cdot \ldots \cdot a$ *Examples:* $3^4 = 3 \cdot 3 \cdot 3 \cdot 3$ or $5^3 = 5 \cdot 5 \cdot 5 = 125$

            n times

(ii) $a^2 = a \times a$ *Examples:* $4^2 = 4 \times 4 = 16$ or $7^2 = 7 \times 7 = 49$

(iii) $a^3 = a \cdot a \cdot a$ *Example:* $2^3 = 2 \cdot 2 \cdot 2 = 8$

Exercise Set X – 1

Perform the operations as indicated.

1. $7 + 2 - 4 + 3 =$ **2.** $5 \times 3 \times 6 =$

3. $2^2 + (3 + 4) - 5 + 1 =$ **4.** $(3 \times 7) \times 2 + 5 =$

5. $2\left[14 - 3(5 - 2)\right]^2 + 2^2 =$ **6.** $4 \times 3 \div 2 \times 3 =$

7. $5(4 \times 6) =$ **8.** $(4 + 3) \times \dfrac{1}{7} =$

Evaluate.

Example: $2 + x - 3y$ where $x = 5, y = 2$

$$2 + (5) - 3(2)$$
$$2 + 5 - 6 = 1$$

9. $x + 7y - 10$ $x = 8, y = 3$

10. $a + 2b + 3c$ $a = 2, b = 3, c = 5$

11. $26 - 3x + 5$ $x = 7$

12. $35 + 3x - 10 + 2y$ $x = 2, y = 7$

13. $2(x + 5) - x^2$ $x = 3$

14. $x^2 - 2y + 3(5 - x)$ $x = 4, y = 3$

You can see that the last group of problems are similar to the previous ones except for the variables within the problem. In all of the problems in exercise set VII – 1, you determined the value of the given expression, substituting given values for variables where directed.

Solving Simple Equations

The basic idea to solving equations involves replacing an equation by an equivalent, but simpler one, and continuing that process until the simplest equation of all appears: $x =$ some number. There are four basic one-step equations that typically occur just before that final solution. Note that whatever happens on one side of an equation, the exact same thing must occur on the other side as well. Otherwise, they won't be equivalent equations and any answer will be incorrect.

Addition

$$\begin{array}{r} x + 5 = 8 \\ -5 \quad -5 \\ \hline x = 3 \end{array}$$

Undo the addition by subtraction.

Subtraction

$$\begin{array}{r} x - 4 = 2 \\ +4 \quad +4 \\ \hline x = 6 \end{array}$$

Undo the subtraction by adding.

Multiplication

$6x = 24$

$\dfrac{6x}{6} = \dfrac{24}{6}$

$1x = 4$
_____

$x = 4$

Undo the multiplication by using division. Note any number divided by itself is 1 and recall the use of unity regarding the rules.

Division

$x \div 5 = 40$

$\underline{\times 5 \quad \times 5}$

$x = 200$

Undo division by multiplying

Examples: (i) $x - 11 = 14$

$\underline{+11 \quad +11}$

$x = 25$

(ii) $\dfrac{x}{6} = 8$

$\underline{\times 6 \quad \times 6}$

$x = 48$

Practice Set X – 2

Solve these one-step equations.

1. $x + 14 = 39$ **2.** $x - 14 = 9$ **3.** $8x = 37$ **4.** $14 = 8x$

5. $27 - x = 8$ **6.** $x \div 6 = 48$ **7.** $\dfrac{x}{9} = 16$ **8.** $136 - x = 49$

More complicated equations simply require additional steps. The key is to create simpler equations until you find the answer. If you do something to an equation, it should then be simpler. If not, you probably are taking the wrong direction to solve.

One situation frequently encountered involves variables (letters) on both sides of the equation. Remember, your goal is to get variables on one side and numbers on the other. Here are some simple rules that may help when you encounter equations with variables on both sides.

There are three situations. (i) variables occur on both sides of an equation and both variables are positive. In that case subtract the smaller one from the larger. Be sure to do the same thing to both sides of the equation (as shown.)

Examples:

(i) $8x + 7 = 3x - 2$ Subtract the smaller from both sides of the equation.

$$\underline{-3x \qquad -3x}$$

$5x + 7 = -2$ Now, variables are only on one side. Undo the addition

$$\underline{-7 \quad -7}$$ by subtracting 7 from both sides. Watch signs!

$5x = -9$

$x = -\dfrac{9}{5} = -1\dfrac{4}{5}$ Here's a one-step equation. Undo the multiplication by dividing both sides by 5. Simplify, if necessary.

(ii) $11x - 5 = 8x + 9$ Subtract the smaller 8x from the

$$\underline{-8x \qquad -8x}$$ larger 11x. Do same on both sides.

$3x - 5 = +9$ Notice the equation has gotten

$$\underline{+5 \quad +5}$$ simpler. You must be doing something

$3x \ = \ 14$ right! Add 5 to both sides

$\dfrac{3x}{3} = \dfrac{14}{3}$ Undo the multiplication of three by the variable by dividing both sides by 3.

$x = \dfrac{14}{3} = 4\dfrac{2}{3}$ Simplify.

In this next situation, the variable on one side of the equation is negative and the same variable on the other side is positive. In this case, add the negative to both sides.

Examples:

(i) $9x - 7 = -4x + 5$

$\underline{+4x \qquad + 4x}$

$13x - 7 = 5$

$\underline{\quad + 7 \quad + 7}$

$13x = 12$

$x = \dfrac{12}{13}$

This eliminates the negative version of the variable as well as getting all the letters on one side of the equation.

(ii) $-11x - 7 = 3x + 4$

$\underline{+11x \qquad + 11x}$

$-7 = 14x + 4$

$\underline{-4 = \qquad - 4}$

$-11 = 14x$

$x = -\dfrac{11}{14}$

Eliminating variables in this manner will yield a positive signed variable.

Write simpler equations until solution found.

In our final example, we have the case where the variables on both sides of the equation are negatively signed. In this case, add the larger (in absolute value) to achieve a positive variable.

Examples:

(i)

$-5x - 7 = -8x + 2$

$\underline{+8x \qquad + 8x}$

$3x - 7 = 2$

$\underline{\quad + 7 \quad + 7}$

$3x = 9$

$x = 3$

This method not only eliminates the variable from one side of the equation, but also eliminates the negatively signed variable.

Continue to simplify and solve as usual.

(ii) $-7x - 6 = -6x - 7$ What may appear
             $\underline{+7x\qquad\ \ + 7x}$ difficult, can be simple
             $-6 = x - 7$ to solve.
             $\underline{+7\qquad + 7}$
             $1 = x$

Notice that multiple–step equations snuck into the previous examples. This demonstrates that no matter how complicated the problem may first appear, apply solution techniques consistently, getting simpler and simpler equations until the answer is determined.

Practice Set X – 3
   Solve.

1. $3x + 7 = 94$ **2.** $8 - 4x = 12x$ **3.** $6x - 5 = 8x + 2$

4. $x + 15 = -3x - 19$ **5.** $\dfrac{2x}{7} + 6 = 34$ **6.** $12 = 7x - 2$

7. $-5x + 8 = -7x - 9$ **8.** $3(x + 1) = -2x + 13$ **9.** $7x - 1 = -8$

10. $-14x - 11 = -11x - 14$ **11.** $3 + 8x = 47$ **12.** $-5 - 7x = 3x + 25$

13. $64 + 3x = 18 + 7x$ **14.** $-16x + 27 = -42x + 19$ **15.** $\dfrac{x}{13} = 6$

To solve linear equations in one variable:

      1. Remove any grouping symbols using the distributive or associative properties.

      2. Add like terms on the left–hand side of the equation.

      3. Add like terms on the right–hand side of the equation.

      4. Eliminate the variables from one side of the equation.

      5. Eliminate the constants from the other side of the equation.

      6. Divide by the coefficient of the variable, if any.

Examples: (i)

$$2(x+7) + 3x = 15 - 4(x+2)$$

Remove parenthesis using the distributive property.

$$2x + 14 + 3x = 15 - 4x - 8$$
$$5x + 14 = 7 - 4x$$

Combine like terms on each side of the equation.

$$9x + 14 = 7$$

Eliminate variables from one side of the equation.

$$9x = 7 - 14$$
$$9x = -7$$

Constants all combined on the side opposite the variables.

$$\frac{9x}{9} = \frac{-7}{9}$$
$$x = -\frac{7}{9}$$

Divide by the coefficient of the variable.

(ii) $5x + 3(x-4) + 17 = -2x + 4(x+7)$

$$5x + 3x - 12 + 17 = -2x + 4x + 28$$
$$8x + 5 = 2x + 28$$
$$6x + 5 = 28$$
$$6x = 23$$
$$x = \frac{23}{6} = 3\frac{5}{6}$$

Eliminate grouping symbols; combine like terms. Get all variables on one side of the equation and constants on the other. Divide by the coefficient of the variable.

Practice Set X – 4

Solve.

1. $15 + 2(x - 5) + 7x = 5x + 3(x - 2)$ 2. $7(x + 1) = 4(x - 2) + 4x$

3. $2x + 21 = 3\left[4 - 5(x - 1)\right]$ 4. $18(x - 1) = 7(x + 2) + 6$

5. $38 + 6x - 2(x - 4) = 2x + 5$ 6. $42 = 7(x + 3)$

7. $20 - 2x + 2(x + 1) = 7x + 5$ 8. $16 - 8x + 5(x + 3) = 9x - 7$

9. $-3x + 7(3 + x) = 2(8 - x) + 9$ 10. $26 - (x + 1) + 5x = -7 - 2(3 + x)$

Inequalities

Inequalities indicate equations that are unbalanced on one side. That is, one side is greater than, indicated $>$, or is less than, indicated $<$. For a simple illustration, look to the number line.

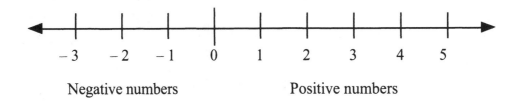

Negative numbers   Positive numbers

Numbers get larger as you move farther to the right and get smaller as you move left. Numbers to the left of zero are negative numbers. They get smaller and smaller further left along the number line. You can see (and you know) that 5 is larger than 2. Algebraically, we say $5 > 2$. In fact, we can even say that $5 \geq 2$. Read as 5 is greater than or equal to 2. It is the *or* part of this statement that makes the entire statement true.

Saying $x \geq 2$, means that x can be 2 or any number that is greater than 2, like 7, or 15, or $2\frac{1}{2}$, or 3.19. Any one of these values, and infinitely more, will make the statement true.

To solve an inequality, use the same techniques and all the same rules as used to solve equations. There is one notable exception. If, during the course of finding the solution, you multiply or divide the inequality by a negative number, you must reverse the inequality sign.

Examples: (i) $x + 2 > 17$ As for an equation, subtract
                       $\underline{-2\ \ -2}$ two from each side.

                       $x > 15$
                                          The solution, x is greater than 15 means x can take on any value as long as it is not 15 or less.

(ii) $3x - 5 > 22$

$\underline{+5 \quad +5}$ Add five to both sides.

$3x > 27$

$\dfrac{3}{3}x > \dfrac{27}{3}$ Divide both sides by 3 to isolate the variable x.

$x > 9$

The solution for x is any number greater than 9.

(iii) $4x + 1 \leq 57$ Like an equation, subtract one from each side of the inequality.

$\underline{-1 \quad -1}$

$4x \leq 56$

$\dfrac{4x}{4} \leq \dfrac{56}{4}$ Undo the multiplication, by dividing by 4 on each side of the inequality and simplify.

$x \leq 14$

The solution, x is less than or equal to 14, indicates that any number that is 14 or less satisfies.

Practice Set X – 5

Solve the inequality.

1. $x + 5 \geq 23$ 2. $x - 7 < 28$ 3. $2x + 1 > 15$

4. $5x - 6 \geq 48$ 5. $7x + 10 \leq 65$ 6. $8x - 3 \leq 15$

7. $x - 20 > 12$ 8. $3x - 5 < 28$ 9. $6x + 7 \geq 49$

Remember, if you multiply or divide an inequality by a negative number, then you must reverse the inequality sign.

Examples: *(i)* $7 - 2x > 11$ As with an equation, undo the positive 7 by subtracting 7 from both sides of the inequality.

$$\underline{-7 \qquad -7}$$

$$-2x > 4$$

$$\frac{-2x}{-2} \; ? \; \frac{4}{-2}$$ To isolate the variable, we must undo the multiplication by dividing by a negative two. This applies to both sides of the inequality.

$$x < -2$$ Since the solution required division by a negative number, the inequality sign is affected. The rule applies – reverse the inequality sign to get the solution x is any number less than a negative 2.

(ii) $-3x + 5 \leq 38$ Subtract 5 from both sides of the inequality.

$$\underline{-5 \quad -5}$$

$$-3x \leq 33$$ Divide by a negative three to get x by itself. Do this on both sides of the inequality and simplify.

$$\frac{-3x}{-3} \; ? \; \frac{33}{-3}$$

$$x \geq -11$$ Reverse the original inequality sign. Include the "or equal to" part, as shown.

(iii) $21 - 5x < -26$ Undo the positive 21 by subtraction.

$$\underline{-21 \qquad -21}$$

$$-5x < -47$$ The result is a negative number multiplied with the variable. Undo by division, using negative five. This division by a negative number will affect the inequality sign.

$$\frac{-5x}{-5} \; ? \; \frac{-47}{-5}$$

$$x > \frac{47}{5} \; or \; x > 9\frac{2}{5} \; or \; x > 9.4$$

Simplify the solution. Note the reversed inequality sign. The answer should be simplified using common or decimal fractions.

Practice Set X – 6

Solve the inequality.

1. $2x - 3 > 7$ **2.** $4x + 5 < 15$ **3.** $3x + 6 < 10$

4. $7x + 8 > 15$ **5.** $2x + 7 > 30$ **6.** $12 - 5x < 67$

7. $3x + 6 < -3$ **8.** $6 - 4x > 14$ **9.** $8x - 4 < 1$

10. $2(x + 1) - 1 > 9$ **11.** $5(x + 1) - 1 \geq 0$ **12.** $2(2x + 3) - 2 \leq 6$

Applications

1. You need a rental car for business. You have two plans from which to choose. One rental car company charges \$25 per day and \$.10 per mile for a car. The other company charges \$35 per day and \$.08 per mile. Determine the number of miles necessary for the cost of the two plans to equal. If you expect to drive 720 miles, which plan is less expensive.

2. Two health care plans are being offered. One has copayments of $15 per doctor visit and $350 deductible. The other plan has $10 copayments with $500 deductible. According to your records, last year you made 8 visits to your doctor and were charged a total of $720 including an annual physical. Which plan should you choose for this year, if you anticipate no major changes in your health?

3. A healthy body temperature should be within 1.5 degrees of a standard normal temperature of 98.6° F. A formula which models this temperature range is $|t - 98.6| \leq 1.5$. Is a temperature of 101°F healthy? How about 97°F? Is 100°F too high a temperature?

4. Body Mass Index (BMI) is one indicator used to measure obesity. A formula for computing the BMI is to divide the patient's weight in kilograms by their height in meters squared. Determine the BMI for the following three patients. If necessary, round to the nearest tenth.

a. Male weighing 86.5 kilograms and 1.83 m tall.

b. Female who is 1.55 m in height in and weighs 48 kg.

c. A 12-year old child who weighs 31 kg and is 140 cm tall.

5. Insulin is typically packaged in 10 cc vials with the concentration of units/cc listed on the label. The concentration can vary, so care must be taken to use the correct dosage. Suppose a patient uses a form of insulin in 10 cc vials with 100 units of insulin per ml. If the patient requires 300 units, how many cc's will be administered?

Suppose the patient was going on a 2 week trip. Their prior use indicated that they used 500 units per day, on average. What is the minimum number of vials they should travel with?

6. A bottle of disinfectant soap contains 118 ml. If a medical care worker typically uses 8 ml for each hand washing, how many times can it be used?

7. An employee earned $575 for a 44 hour week. The employee earns time–and–a–half for hours worked over 40. What is the employees regular hourly wage?

Graphs and Graphing Techniques

A graph is a visual means of presenting numerical data to show relationships between one set of numbers and another. Graphs of data sometimes must be prepared by the technician. Usually the graph will have a vertical axis called the *y* axis (ordinate) and a horizontal axis called the *x* axis (abscissa).

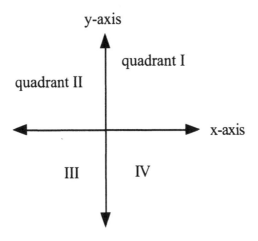

A two dimensional rectangular graph has four quadrants. The center point is called the origin and is labeled (0, 0). Any point in the plane, that is, on the graph is denoted with an *ordered* pair of numbers (x, y) which tell the location of that particular point. It is called an ordered pair since the order matters. The first number denotes movement left and right in line with the x–axis; the second number gives the vertical movement.

Each axis is divided into the desired units. These units describe some term of the experiment which can be measured. An example might be light absorbed by a solution measured on one axis and concentration of the solution measured on the other axis. Heart rate, respiration, or pulse over time might be another example, as well as average weight versus age or height.

Generally, it makes no difference which item of interest is plotted on the x–axis and which is plotted on the y–axis. The divisions are spaced and numbered according to a convenient measurement. In the example shown, time is measured in minutes and temperature in degrees Celsius. The time scale could have been shown in seconds but the graph would have been larger (much more "spread out"). A scale should be chosen relative to the data being recorded and in such a way as to facilitate or enhance the visual information being conveyed. In this case, the time measurement is on the x–axis and temperature scale is on the y–axis.

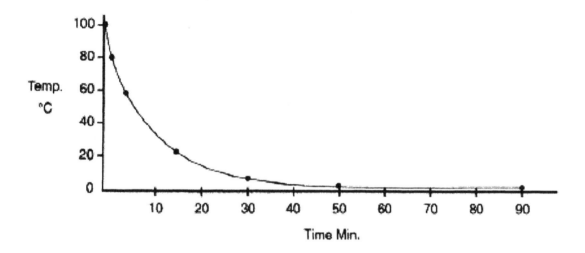

The numbers for the upper limit should be equal to or slightly larger than the largest data value. You would not select 80 minutes when the last point turned out to be at 90 minutes since this would eliminate some of the data. The lower limit, likewise, must be less than or equal to the lowest value. In many cases the lowest value is zero. But be aware of distorted (truncated) graphs which do not start at zero. However, many legitimate graphs do start at some number other than zero.

Examples of graphs

(i) **ECG** graphs – top view indicates interference occurred during the recording. The bottom view is a standard result.

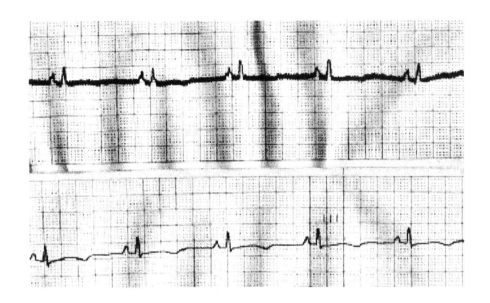

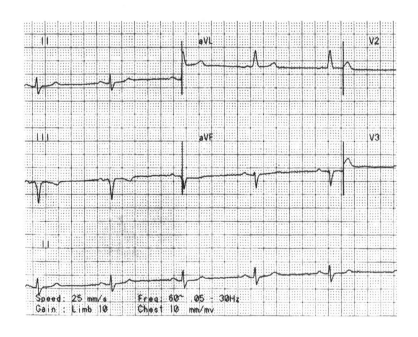

(ii)   Chart showing respiration rate and pulse rate recorded over time

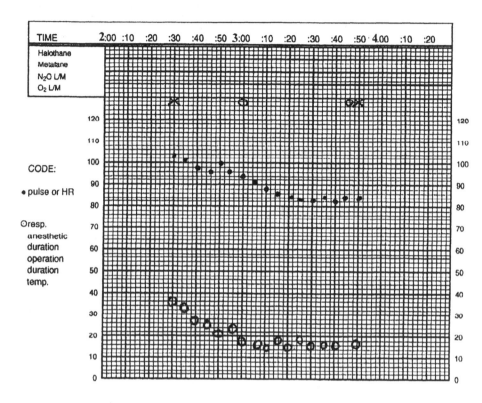

(iii)   Blood and Urine chemistries are usually line graphs.

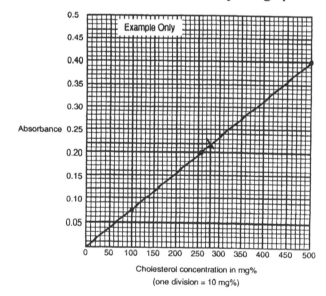

Plotting data on the graph can show changes, trends, and relative quantities.

The x-axis is designated one variable (time, in this example) while the vertical y-axis is designated as another variable (heart rate). Label each axis with the type of measurement such as time, rate and temperature and also with the respective units (sec, min, beats per min, degrees C.)

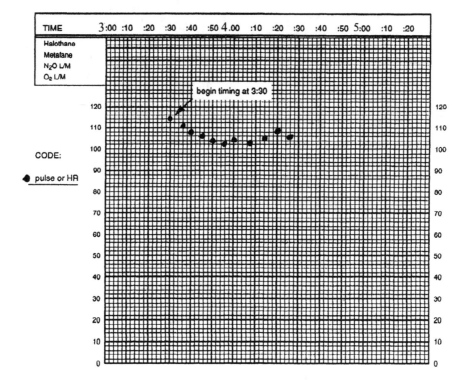

Plotting the graph

The most common uses of graphs for the technician involves Quadrant I or Quadrants I and IV

Examples:

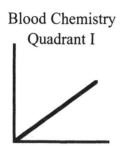

Blood Chemistry
Quadrant I

Quadrants I & IV – ECG

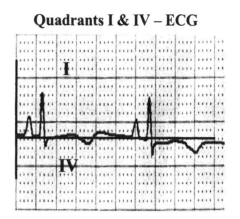

Plotting rectangular coordinates

Plotting a graph

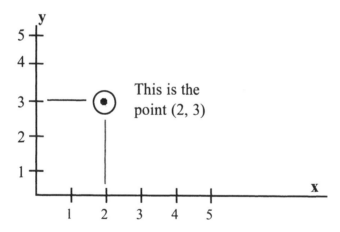

The first value in the ordered pair (2) denotes the distance in line with the *x*-axis; the second value of the ordered pair (3) denotes the distance vertically in line with the *y*-axis. The point is plotted where the two corresponding imaginary lines meet.

An example best illustrates how to determine where points on graphs should be placed. In this example, use 0.30 A, which is a measure of the quantity of light absorbed and a concentration of the solution of 3%.

Start at zero (0) and proceeds 3 units to the right along the x-axis. This corresponds to the 3% concentrate. Next, proceed vertically for 3 units which corresponds to 0.30 on the scale of the y-axis. At this point, make a dot (as shown.) The procedure could have been reversed with no effect on the results. Going up 3 units and then over 3 units will yield the same point on the graph.

Concentration (%)

Other known or observed values may be plotted on the same graph. As in the graph example above, the following points are plotted in the same manner. Those points are joined with a straight line.

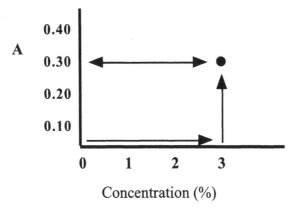

A	% Conc
0.1	1
0.2	2
0.3	3
0.4	4
0.5	5

Concentration (%)

A straight line is composed of points derived from known values and plotted relative to both the x – and y – axes.

Many solutions have known concentrations. The absorbency of light, denoted A, by a solution, is determined using a spectrophotometer. These values can then be plotted on a graph and a line drawn through the points. The graph as a visual reference then shows a positive relationship between the variables. As the concentration of the solution increases, the amount of light absorbed also increases.

Another use for the graph is that once a relationship is shown and plotted, the line can be used to find corresponding concentrations given the amount of light absorbed. Or, if it is known how much light is absorbed by a solution, the concentration can be determined. Using the graph in this manner saves the trouble of having to always measure every single item.

Example: Using the given information, plot a standard curve of concentration at absorbency (A).

Concentration v Absorbency

Conc (%)	A
1	0.05
2	0.10
3	0.15
4	0.20
5	0.25

Determining values from an unknown:

Once the graph has been plotted, it can be used to determine concentrations of other solutions by measuring Absorbency using a spectrophotometer.

Using the standard curve, the concentration of an unknown solution is placed in a spectrophotometer and the absorbency is determined. On the graph shown below, (1) go up the y-axis (A) until that value is reached. (2) Then proceed parallel to the x-axis (concentration) until the standard curve is intersected. (3) Now drop vertically to the x-axis to (4) read the corresponding concentration of the solution.

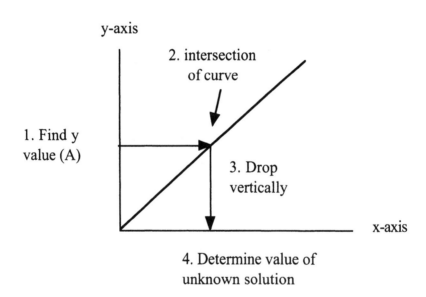

Practice Set 10 – 7

1. Using the given chart of concentration v Absorbency (A), plot the points, draw a line and determine the concentrations for the given absorbencies to complete the table that follows.

<u>A</u>	<u>Concentration (mg%)</u>
0.09	100
0.23	260
0.45	500

Unknown Solution	A	Concentration
A	0.16	_____
B	0.22	_____
C	0.15	_____
D	0.09	_____
E	0.12	_____
F	0.24	_____

2. Given the following graph and values, interpolate for cholesterol levels to complete the chart that follows.

Conc (%)	A
1	0.05
2	0.10
3	0.15
4	0.20
5	0.25

Sample	Absorbency	concentration %
A	0.10	_____
B	0.20	_____
C	0.30	_____
D	0.35	_____
E	0.27	_____
F	0.18	_____

Plotting graphs using quadrants I and IV such as for an EKG.

All values along the x-axis are positive. However, y values may be positive or negative. Those y values that lie above the x-axis are positive (in quadrant I) and those below the x-axis (in quadrant IV) are negative.

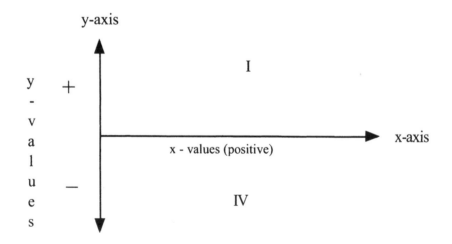

3. Recall that coordinates for a point are given as an ordered pair, (x, y). On the following graph, find the (x. y) ordered pair values for each lettered point on the graph.

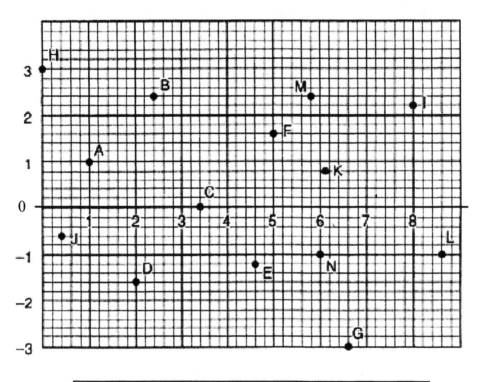

	(x, y)		(x, y)
A		H	
B		I	
C		J	
D		K	
E		L	
F		M	
G		N	

Unit IV

Chapter 11
Dosage and Concentration Applications
Using Ratios and Proportions

Understanding and solving word problems involves some of the most critical skills a professional can learn. We communicate both orally and with the written word as we work together in an office or clinic. The doctor who asks for 3 cc of atropine for an injection, for instance, trusts the nurse to supply exactly that. The calculation of dosages is a critical area — it must be done quickly and accurately. The dosage is the required amount to administer for a particular patient for a specific result. The concentration is the potency of the medicine – the amount of medicine, or active ingredient, in a given volume or per tablet.

When solving word problems, there are several principles that are useful:
- Decide what is being asked. What is needed for the result?
- Catalog the information given - write it down!
- Determine the ratio and proportions needed, including the units.

Example: A dose of sodium pentobarbital is needed for a 125 pound patient. The dosage provided on the label is 1 cc per 25 pounds of body weight.

1. What is needed? – the amount to administer to the patient is x cc.

2. Known information: dosage of $\dfrac{1\,cc}{25\,lbs}$; weight of patient – 125 pounds.

3. Determine the appropriate proportion: $\dfrac{X\,cc}{125\,lbs} = \dfrac{1\,cc}{25\,lbs}$

4. Solve: $\dfrac{X\,cc}{125\,lbs} = \dfrac{1\,cc}{25\,lbs}$ The lbs units cancel; 25 divides evenly into 125

$$X\,cc = \dfrac{\overset{5}{\cancel{125\,lbs}} \times 1\,cc}{\underset{1}{\cancel{25\,lbs}}}$$

$$X = 5\,cc$$

The correct dosage for the 125 pound patient is 5 cc.

Using dimensional analysis:

$$\frac{\overset{5}{\cancel{125\ \cancel{lbs}}}}{\underset{1}{\cancel{25\ \cancel{lbs}}}} \cdot \frac{1\ cc}{} = 5\ cc$$

Pound units cancel and 25 divides into 125 evenly ("cancels")

(ii) A 210 pound patient is prescribed a dosage of medicine of 100 mg per 10 pounds Body Weight (B.W.). How many milligrams should be administered?

$$\frac{\overset{21}{\cancel{210\ lbs}}}{\underset{1}{\cancel{10\ lbs}}} \cdot \frac{100\ mg}{} = 2100\ mg$$

Pounds units cancel leaving the result in milligrams. Numbers cancel as in fractions.

Practice Set XI – 1

Solve the following problems.

1. How much Procainamide is needed for an 80 kg adult if the dosage is 5 mg per kilogram of body weight?

2. How much Procainamide would be necessary if the patient weighed 50 kg?

3. A dispyramide medication is prescribed at doses of 6 – 15 milligrams per kilogram body weight (B.W.) per day.

    a. How many milligrams are necessary to dose a 60 kg adult with the maximum concentration?

    b. How many mg to provide the minimum dosage to a 34 kg adolescent?

4. How much anticoagulant is necessary for a 150 pound patient if the dosage is 15 cc per 10 pounds B.W.?

5. If a 210 lb patient requires 25 cc of medication, how many cc will a 175 lb patient require if the same ratio holds?

Some medicines in the clinic are prescribed in milligrams per pound of body weight, yet they're packaged in milligrams per cc. To compute the proper dosage requires multiple steps:

- calculate the number of mg to be given for a particular weight of patient
- calculate the number of cc which contains the number of mg computed

Example: An anesthetic is given at the dosage of 15 mg per 10 lb body weight. It is packaged in vials at a concentration of 100 mg per 1 cc. How many cc should be given to a 127 lb (*or* 57.73 kg) patient?

(i) Determine the amount of medication in mg based upon the 127 lb patient.

$$\frac{x}{127\ lbs} = \frac{15\ mg}{10\ lbs} \quad \text{cross-multiply and simplify}$$

$$x = \frac{127\ lbs \times 15\ mg}{10\ lbs} \quad \text{note the lbs units cancel}$$

$$x = 190.5\ mg$$

(ii) This gives the amount of medicine necessary. Determine the cc equivalent.

$$\frac{x}{190.5\ mg} = \frac{1\ cc}{100\ mg} \qquad \begin{array}{l}\text{solve the proportion by}\\ \text{cross-multiplying and}\\ \text{simplifying}\end{array}$$

$$x = \frac{190.5\ mg \times 1\ cc}{100\ mg}$$

$$x = 1.905\ cc\ or\ 1.91\ cc \qquad \begin{array}{l}\text{Round to nearest}\\ \text{hundredth cc}\end{array}$$

Same problem using dimensional analysis.

$$\frac{127\ lbs}{} \left| \frac{15\ mg}{10\ lb} \right| \frac{1\ cc}{100\ mg} = \frac{1905\ cc}{1000} = 1.905\ cc = 1.91\ cc$$

Some problems may have the additional step requiring a change in units from body weight in pounds to weight in kilograms, or vice versa. Once more – the previous problem using dimensional analysis and including the conversion from weight in kilograms to weigh in pounds.

$$\frac{57.73 \text{ kg} \mid 2.2 \text{ lb} \mid 15 \text{ mg} \mid 1 \text{ cc}}{\mid 1 \text{ kg} \mid 10 \text{ lb} \mid 100 \text{ mg}} = \frac{1905.09 \text{ } cc}{1000} = 1.91 \, cc$$

Practice Set XI – 2

1. How many cc of an antibiotic should be administered to a 170 pound patient when the doctor has prescribed a dosage of 0.5 mg per pound of body weight? The anesthetic is packaged in a concentration of 10 mg per 1 cc.

2. A phenobarbital preparation is given to a patient at the rate of 0.3 mg per pound of body weight. The patient weighs 142 pounds. The concentration is 5 mg per cc. How many cc should be administered?

3. The same preparation is prescribed in a dosage of 0.5 mg / lb. for a 185 pound patient. How many cc are necessary if the concentration is 5 mg per cc?

4. A Sulfa drug is to be given to a 130 pound patient at the rate of 2.5 mg per lb. How many cc are necessary if the concentration is 200 mg per cc?

5. Morphine has been prescribed at the rate of 0.1 mg per kg B.W. for a 90 kilogram patient. The concentration is 10 mg per cc. How many cc should be administered?

6. A phenobarbital preparation is prescribed for pediatric use at 1 to 3 milligrams per kilogram of B.W.. A child weighing 88 pounds would receive how many milligrams for a minimum dosage? How many mg for the maximum dosage?

7. The same phenobarbital preparation is prescribed for adults at 15 to 20 milligrams per kilogram of B.W.. What is the maximum amount an adult who weighs 198 pounds? (b) How much is the minimum dosage for a 126 pound female patient?

8. A phenobarbital preparation is available in 15 mg, 30 mg, 100 mg and 5000 mg tablets. For the patients in problem **7**, weighing 198 lbs and 126 lbs, how many tablets and of what size should be dispensed to achieve the closest possible result to the doses computed and without splitting any tablets?

9.   **a.** A 150 pound patient receives 8,000 units of a sodium anticoagulant in concentrated solution delivered by injection every 8 hours. How many units would be expected to be administered over a 6 day recovery period?

        b. For continuous I.V. infusion, 20,000 to 40,000 units every 24 hours is prescribed. How many 1000 ml bags of sodium chloride solution at 8 units/ml would be needed for a maximum dosage?

        10. A Hydrochloric topical anesthetic used for children is prescribed after considering a variety of factors such as age, weight and body mass type. The maximum dosage for a child of 5 to 7 years and weighing 50 pounds should not exceed 75 to 100 mg. Determine the proper dosage for a 7 year old child weighing 42 pounds if the dosage is 4.5 mg per kilogram of body weight.

Practice Set XI – 3

    1. Procainamide is prescribed at 50 mg per kilogram of Body Weight.

        a. How many mg are needed for a 80 kg adult?

        b. How many milligrams are necessary to treat a 110 lb adult female?

2. A disopyramide medication treatment is prescribed at 6 – 15 milligrams per kilogram B.W. per day.

        a. How many milligrams would be necessary to dose a 132 lb adult with the maximum concentration? How much is needed for a 3 day course of treatment?

        b. How many milligrams to provide the minimum dosage to a 50 kilogram adolescent? How many milligrams are necessary for 5 days of treatment?

3. Disopyramide is available in 150 mg, 250 mg and 450 mg capsules.

        a. How many capsules are necessary to treat the 132 pound adult in (**2a**) for one day? How many capsules, of which type, for a 6 day course of treatment?

        b. How many capsules, of which type, should be dispensed to treat the 50 kg adolescent patient (in problem **2b**) for 10 days?

4. An amakin sulfate preparation is prescribed at the rate of 15 mg per kg of B.W.

        a. How much is necessary for a 61 kg patient?

        b. How many for an adult male weighing 176 pounds?

5. A chlorpromazine tranquilizer can be used for children at $1/4$ mg per pound B.W. How much should be administered to a 100 pound child? The medication is available in 25 mg, 50 mg, and 100 mg tablets. Which tablet would be most appropriate to administer?

6. An amoxicillin preparation prescribed for a mild infection can be delivered in doses of 25 milligrams per kilogram body weight every 12 hours; or at 20 mg/kg for dosing every 8 hours.

        a. Determine the appropriate dosage for a patient weighing 57 kilos with doses
           i. every 8 hours

           ii. every 12 hours

        b. Calculate the dosage to be administered every 12 hours to a male patient who weighs 132 pounds.

7. The amoxicillin solution can be prescribed for a moderate to severe condition in the lower respiratory tract at the dosage of 45 mg/kg given every 12 hours or 40 mg/kg every 8 hours.

        a. Determine the appropriate dosage for a 60 kilogram patient to be given:
           i. every 8 hours

           ii. every 12 hours

        b. Determine the dosage for a 132 pound patient who will receive their medication every 12 hours.

8. For a narcotic overdose, a naloxone injection may be indicated. For children this dosage is 0.01 mg per kg of B. W. How much should be administered for an adolescent weighing 98 pounds?

9. A bleomycin sulfate preparation is injected weekly to combat squamous cell carcinoma. The usual dose is $1/4$ to $1/2$ units per kilogram. For an adult patient who weighs 187 pounds, determine the correct dosage for a maximum treatment.

10. A buterol hydrochloric inhalation solution has a concentration of 0.63 mg per 3 ml. The dosage is 2 mg per 10 pounds B.W. For a child weighing 62 pounds, determine the correct milligram dosage and the milliliter amount to be administered.

Occasionally, an order may involve an initial injection of the dose followed by the remainder some time, say 15 minutes, later. In this case, compute the total dosage required. Determine the appropriate initial dose for the patient. Find the amount that remains. Determine the points on the syringe that correspond to the correct administration of the medicine.

Example: A certain anesthetic drug is ordered to be administered to an adolescent weighing 35 kilograms. The dosage rate is 0.5 cc per 10 lb B.W.

a. What is the total amount to be administered?

$$\frac{35 \, \cancel{kg} \mid 2.2 \, \cancel{lb} \mid 0.5 \, cc}{\mid 1 \, \cancel{kg} \mid 10 \, \cancel{lb \, BW}} = 11 \, cc$$

b. So any adverse reaction can be noted, only 60% is to be given immediately, with the remainder injected after 15 minutes. How many cc will initially be discharged?

$$11 \, cc \times 60\% = 11 \times 0.60 = 6.6 \, cc$$

c. Shown is a 12 cc syringe. Assume that the syringe is filled with the amount calculated in **a**. Indicate by an arrow (↓) on the syringe where this would be.

Indicate using a double arrow (⇓) the point where the medication would be discharged to administer the initial 60%.

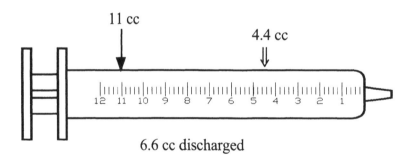

6.6 cc discharged

Note that 6.6 cc initially injected implies the plunger should move from 11 cc to 4.4 cc. That is, subtract the amount to be injected at first from the total.

Practice Set XI – 4

1. A pentobarbital concentration is administered to an adolescent weighing 54.5 kilograms. The dosage rate is 1 cc per 15 lb B.W.

    a. What is the total amount to be administered (to nearest tenth)?

    b. So any adverse reaction can be noted, only 60% is to be given immediately, with the remainder injected after 15 minutes. How many cc will initially be discharged?

    c. Shown is a 12 cc syringe. Assume that the syringe is filled with the amount calculated in **a**. Indicate by an arrow (⬇) on the syringe where this would be.

Indicate using a double arrow (⇓) the point where the medication would be discharged to administer the initial 60%.

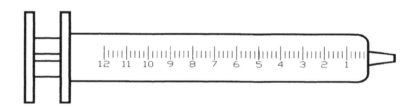

2. A similar barbital medication is to be administered to a 51 kilogram female patient. The dosage is 1 cc per 15 lb.

    a. What is the total amount needed (to nearest tenth)?

    b. If 60% is administered initially, How many cc are needed?

c. Shown is a 12 cc syringe. Assume that the syringe is filled with the amount calculated in (i). Indicate by an arrow (↓) on the syringe where this would be.

Indicate using a double arrow (⇓) the point where the medication would be discharged to administer the initial 60%.

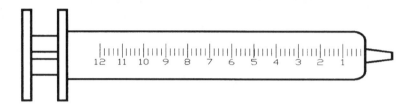

3. The same medication is prescribed for an adult male who weighs 79.5 kilograms. The dosage is 1 cc per 25 lb.

    a. What is the total amount of the prescribed dose (to nearest tenth)?

    b. 60% is to be administered initially. How many cc will that take?

    c. Shown is a 12 cc syringe. Assume that the syringe is filled with the amount calculated in (i). Indicate by an arrow (↓) on the syringe where this would be.

Indicate using a double arrow (⇓) the point where the medication would be discharged to administer the initial 60%.

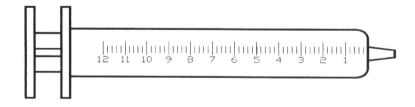

Solutions that are prepared from concentrations can be made by determining the value of the percent of concentration and changing this to grams. Dissolve the appropriate gram amount in water to make 100 ml of the correct concentration of the needed solution.

Review of terms

% means parts per 100

grams% means grams per 100 ml

Thus, the term % can represent either grams per 100 ml or ml per 100 ml

Solutions used in practices can be formulated as needed. Dissolving a salt in distilled water, for instance, will make a saline solution. The concentration of the solution determines the amount of chemical necessary.

Solutions typically have a concentration of chemical to water or alcohol. A 10% solution has 10 parts per 100. Practically that means there are 10 grams of say, salt, dissolved in 100 ml of water.

Example: A 0.9% sodium chloride solution is required. Dissolve 0.9 grams of sodium chloride in 100 ml water to make 100 ml of 0.9% solution.

The problem can be more complex if the desired volume is not 100 ml. For example, how much sodium chloride would be needed to prepare only 60 ml of 0.9% solution?

Solve this problem using the same ratio and proportion methods you have been using.

It is known that: $\dfrac{0.9\,g}{100\,ml}$ but what is needed is $\dfrac{?\,g}{60\,ml}$ in order to achieve the correct concentration.

$$\frac{x}{60\,ml} = \frac{0.9g}{100\,ml}$$

cross-multiply and
simplify. The ml
units cancel

$$x = \frac{0.9g \times 60\,ml}{100\,ml}$$

. . . by dimensional analysis

$$x = 0.54g$$

$$\frac{60\,ml}{}\left|\frac{0.9\ g}{100\ ml} = 0.54\ g\right.$$

Thus, 0.54 grams of sodium chloride is needed to make 60 ml of 0.9% solution.

Example: To make 500 ml of a 10% saline solution dissolve
10 grams of salt per 100 ml. Mathematically...

$$\frac{10\ g}{100\ ml} = \frac{x}{500\ ml}$$

Solve this proportion for the missing value.
To make 500 ml of saline solution of the
same 10% concentration, use 50 g of salt.

Using dimensional analysis $$\frac{\overset{5}{500\,ml}}{}\left|\frac{10\ g}{\underset{1}{100\,ml}} = 50\ grams\right.$$

Examples: *(i)* Prepare 600 ml of an 8% saline solution. $8\% \rightarrow \dfrac{8\,g}{100\,ml}$

Form a proportion and solve.

$$\dfrac{8\,g}{100\,ml} = \dfrac{x\,g}{600\,ml} \qquad or \qquad \dfrac{\overset{6}{\cancel{600\,ml}}}{} \left| \dfrac{8\,g}{\underset{1}{\cancel{100\,ml}}} \right. = 48\,g$$

$$x = 48\,g$$

(ii) Make 1000 ml of a 12% solution.

$$12\% = \dfrac{12\,g}{100\,ml}$$

$$\dfrac{12\,g}{100\,ml} = \dfrac{x}{1000\,ml}$$

$$x = 120\,g$$

Example: A solution is composed of 95 ml of water and 5 ml of formalin. Determine the amount of formalin necessary to make 1000 ml of solution of the same concentration.

Total volume of known solution: 95 ml + 5 ml = 100 ml

For every 100 ml of solution, 5 ml of formalin is needed. Written as a proportion:

$$\dfrac{5ml}{100\,ml} = \dfrac{x}{1000ml}$$

$$x = \dfrac{5ml \times 1000\,ml}{100\,ml}$$

$$x = 50\,ml$$

So, 50 ml of formalin is needed to make 1000 ml of the formalin solution.

Practice Set XI – 5

1. How many grams of sodium chloride will be needed to prepare 4000 ml of saline solution at 9% concentration?

2. Prepare 4000 ml of 5% dextrose solution.

3. Prepare 1000 ml of 2.5% dextrose solution.

4. Prepare 500 ml of 10% dextrose solution.

5. Prepare 3000 ml of 5% formalin solution. (Formalin is measured in ml)

6. Prepare 4000 ml of 10% formalin solution.

7. Calculate the amount of each chemical needed to make 600 ml of solution if one gram of Iodine and two grams potassium Iodine is used to make 100 ml of solution.

8. If a solution calls for 2 ml Acetic Acid and 98 ml of H_2O, and 1600 ml of the solution is needed; how much acetic acid should be used?

9. If 1000 ml of a certain solution contains 1.5 g NaCl, how many grams of NaCl are needed to make 1500 ml of the solution?

10. It takes 1 g of mercuric bichloride to make 1200 ml of solution. How many grams of mercuric bichloride would it take to make 750 ml of solution?

11. In making a 2% solution, 16 g of boric acid crystals are dissolved in 800 ml of water. How many grams of boric acid crystals are needed to make 50 ml of 2 % solution?

12. To prepare a certain solution, 1 gram of potassium permanganate crystals is added to 5000 ml of water. How many grams of potassium permanganate crystals should be added to 2000 ml of water to make the same concentration of the solution?

Practice Set XI – 6

For each of the following solutions, determine the number of grams (or ml if liquid) are necessary to:

1. Make a 2500 ml solution of 0.9% saline.

2. Prepare a 525 ml solution of 2% formalin.

3. Prepare 650 ml of 5% formalin solution.

4. Prepare 950 ml of 5% dextrose solution.

5. Make 3250 ml of 10% formalin solution.

6. Make 75 ml of NaCl at 0.9%

7. Prepare 25 ml of 1% alcoholic (in alcohol) solution of phenolphthalein.

8. Make 95 ml of 1% copper sulfate.

9. Make 200 ml of 10% Potassium solution.

10. Prepare 75 ml of a 1% silver nitrate solution.

Calculate the percentage of concentration of a solution by dividing the active ingredient by the total volume of solution.

Examples: *(i)* 320 ml of ethyl alcohol in 500 ml of solution yields a solution of 64% .

$$\frac{320\ ml}{500\ ml} = 0.64 \rightarrow 64\%$$

(ii) 9 grams of saline salt in 50 ml of solution yields $\dfrac{9\ g}{50\ ml} = 0.18 = 18\%$

Ignore units when computing the percentage concentration since percentage is parts per hundred, or, in this case, grams per deciliter.

Calculate the percentage of solution for each of the following.

11. 190 ml of ethyl alcohol in 200 ml of solution.

12. 3.6 g of sodium chloride in 400 ml of water.

13. 4.5 g of copper sulfate in 225 ml of solution.

14. 15 g of glucose in 300 ml of solution.

15. 4.5 g of sodium chloride in 500 ml of solution.

16. 210 ml of isopropyl alcohol in 300 ml of solution.

Practice Set XI – 7

1. An adult with growth hormone deficiency is treated with a drug at the rate of 0.06 mg per kg of B.W.. How many mg are necessary for an 89 kg patient?

2. Kidney infections may be treated with an antibiotic at the rate of 3 mg per kg every 8 hours.

      a. How many mg will be necessary for a 4 day course of treatment for an adult weighing 112 kg?

      b. Up to 5 mg/kg can be administered to seriously infected individuals. How many mg will be needed for the patient under these conditions?

3. A common antibiotic has dosage recommendations of 25 mg/kg every 12 hours or 20 mg/kg every 8 hours. Determine the daily dosage and the amount to be dispensed for each of the following situations.

      a. A 13 year old child weighing 90 pounds is prescribed to receive the medication every 8 hours for 10 days.

      b. A 70 kg adult is prescribed for every 12 hours for 6 days.

      c. An female adolescent is prescribed medication every 12 hours for 8 days. She weighs 99 pounds.

      d. An adult weighing 250 pounds is to be dosed for 7 days every 8 hours.

4. Another common antibiotic can be used for severe respiratory infections at the rate of 45 mg/kg every 12 hours or 40 mg/kg every 8 hours.

a. A 17 year old weighing 134 pounds is ordered to receive the medication every 8 hours for 10 days. How much should he receive each dose? How much per day? How much should be dispensed for the treatment period?

b. A 74 kg adult is ordered to receive medication every 12 hours for 6 days. Determine the amount to be administered per dose. Find the amount that should be taken each day. Find the amount that should be dispensed.

5. Suspected narcotic overdoses can be treated with an injection of medication with a dosage of 0.01 mg/kg B.W. given intravenously. If this dose does not achieve the desired result, a dose of 0.1 mg/kg B.W. may be administered. The medication comes in a concentration of 0.4 mg/ml packaged in 1 ml dosage vials and 1 mg/ml in 2 ml vials.

a. Find the amount a teenager weighing 80 kg should receive for an initial dose. How many vials are needed?

b. After a period of non response, the dose is increased. How much should be administered now? How many vials should be available?

6. Carcinomas of certain types can be treated with an injection of 0.25 to 0.50 units per kg of B.W. given weekly or twice weekly. An adult male with a type of squamous cell carcinoma may receive weekly injections of how many units if he weighs 82.3 kg?

Diluting Solutions and Adjusting Concentrations

In a laboratory, solutions frequently are found in a concentrated form for ease of shipment and storage as well as economies of scale. The concentrated solution is called the *stock* solution. The concentration with which the solution is used can be less than this stock concentration. The result is that the technician must be able to dilute, usually with water, these stock solutions to the desired concentration for a particular use. This is accomplished by mixing some certain amount of stock solution with some amount of *diluent* to achieve the desired result.

For *example:* Isopropyl alcohol (rubbing alcohol) is shipped in concentrations of 100 % alcohol. The most effective concentration to guard against bacteria growth is 70%. The technician must mix the concentrated stock solution (100% alcohol) with water to reach the desired final concentration of 70%.

There are several techniques that can be used to determine the correct mix. We present the most widely used and most practical method. Remember that you *begin with a concentrated solution* and *always dilute* that solution to the desired concentration. A useful formula is provided:

Note: unless otherwise noted, the diluent is water.

$$C_1 \cdot V_1 = C_2 \cdot V_2$$

C_1 is the original concentration of the stock solution

V_1 is the volume of the stock solution used

C_2 is the desired (final) concentration (the one you want to make)

V_2 is the volume of the final concentration

Examples: *(i)* You must prepare 4 L of a 70% isopropyl alcohol solution from the 100 % stock solution. You must determine the volume of stock solution to use as well as the volume of the diluent, water, which must be mixed to achieve 4 liters of total volume.

$$C_1 = 100\% \qquad V_1 = ? \qquad\qquad \text{determine the}$$
$$C_2 = 70\% \qquad V_2 = 4 liters \qquad \text{known information}$$

$$C_1 \cdot V_1 = C_2 \cdot V_2 \qquad\qquad \text{use the formula}$$

$$100\% \times V_1 = 70\% \times 4 liters \qquad \text{substitute the known}$$
$$\text{information into the formula}$$

$$V_1 = \frac{70\% \times 4 liters}{100\%} \qquad \text{cancel the percents; your}$$
$$\text{answer will be in liters}$$

$$V_1 = \frac{280 L}{100}$$

$$V_1 = 2.8 L \quad \text{of 100\% stock solution of}$$
$$\text{isopropyl alcohol is needed}$$

Next determine the volume of diluent (water) to add:

Total volume desired (final volume):	4.0 liters
Volume of (100%) alcohol:	− 2.8 liters
Volume of water needed:	1.2 liters

(ii) You must prepare as much 40% solution isopropyl alcohol as possible from 2.3 L of 100% stock solution. Determine the volume of 40% solution that can be made and the volume of diluent, water, which is used to make the 40% solution.

$C_1 = 100\%$ $V_1 = 2.3$ L
$C_2 = 40\%$ $V_2 = ???$ Determine the known information

$$C_1V_1 = C_2V_2$$

$100\% \cdot 2.3\,L = 40\% \cdot V_2$ Use the formula and
                                              substitute the known
$V_2 = \dfrac{100\% \cdot 2.3\,L}{40\%}$ information. Simplify

$V_2 = 5.75\,Liters$

Total Volume   5.75 liters
          Amount of 100% Alcohol $-$ 2.3 liters
          Volume of water needed   3.45 liters

Practice Set XI – 8

Solve the following problems and determine the amount of diluent.

1. Isopropyl alcohol

<u>stock</u>   <u>desired</u>
$C_1 = 100\%$ $V_1 = ???$ $C_2 = 70\%$ $V_2 = 2.5$ L

2. Ethyl alcohol

$C_1 = 95\%$ $V_1 = ???$
$C_2 = 70\%$ $V_2 = 3$ L

3. Formalin (recall that formalin is a liquid)

$C_1 = 10\%$ $V_1 = ???$
$C_2 = 2\%$ $V_2 = 12$ L

4. For an acetic acid solution

$C_1 = 100\%$ $V_1 = 75$ ml
$C_2 = 2\%$ $V_2 = ???$

5. HCl (hydrochloric acid)

$C_1 = 100\%$ $V_1 = 20$ ml
$C_2 = 1\%$ $V_2 = ???$

6. $NaHCO_3$ (sodium bicarbonate)

$C_1 = 9\%$ $V_1 = ???$
$C_2 = 5\%$ $V_2 = 2500$ ml

7. Isopropyl alcohol

$C_1 = 100\%$ $V_1 = ???$
$C_2 = 70\%$ $V_2 = 3$ L

Practice Set XI – 9   Solve. Also compute the amount of diluent necessary.

1. Isopropyl alcohol

   $C_1 = 100\%$ $C_2 = 70\%$
   $V_1 = \text{???}$ $V_2 = 1 \text{ L}$

2. Ethyl Alcohol

   $C_1 = 95\%$ $C_2 = 70\%$
   $V_1 = \text{???}$ $V_2 = 4 \text{ L}$

3. NaOH

   $C_1 = 30\%$ $C_2 = 5\%$
   $V_1 = 500 \text{ ml}$ $V_2 = \text{???}$

4. Formalin

   $C_1 = 100\%$ $C_2 = 10\%$
   $V_1 = \text{???}$ $V_2 = 20 \text{ L}$

5. Formalin

$C_1 = 10\%$ $C_2 = 2\%$

$V_1 = 1\ L$ $V_2 = \ ???$

6. Hydrogen peroxide

$C_1 = 100\%$ $C_2 = 2\%$

$V_1 = 50\ ml$ $V_2 = \ ???$

Practice Set XI – 10

      Solve each of the following. Determine the volume of stock solution needed *and* the volume of diluent.

1. Prepare 30 L of formalin from a 100% stock solution. How much formalin is needed to make:

     a. a 5% solution?   **b.** a 1% solution?

2. A stock solution of NaCl is 9%. Prepare 6 liters of a 0.9% saline solution. How much stock solution is needed?

3. Ethyl alcohol comes as a 95% stock solution. Prepare:

      a. 6 L of 90%   **b.** 9 L of 70%

4. Sodium hydroxide has been previously prepared in a concentration of 30% (C_1). But you need a concentration of 5% (C_2) and a volume of 1 L (1000 ml) (V_2). How many ml of the 30% solution will you have to use? How much water?

5. Isopropyl alcohol is 100% but the desired strength is 70%. How much of the 100% stock is needed to make 3 gallons of 70% solution?

6. If 20 L of alcohol (100%) was available, how many liters of 70% could you make?

7. 36% HCl needs to be diluted to 1%. Unfortunately there is only 200 ml of HCl left in the lab. How much will this make?

8. Prepare 25 L of a 10% formalin solution from a 100% stock solution. How much of the stock solution do you need? How much water will you use?

9. Further dilute the 10% formalin solution prepared in problem number (**8**) Compute the amount of stock solution to use and the volume of the diluent necessary.

      a. Prepare 500 ml of 5% solution

      b. Make 350 ml of 1% solution.

      On occasion, the technician may need to determine the resultant concentration of solution. For example, 500 ml of 95% alcohol is diluted with 100 ml of water. What is the concentration of the solution?

      Here, the initial concentration, $C_1 = 95\%$ and the initial volume, V_1 is 500 ml. The volume of the solution prepared, V_2 is 600 ml (500 ml of 95% alcohol and 100 ml of water). So, we want to know what C_2, the concentration of the solution that was prepared.

$$C_1V_1 = C_2V_2$$
$$(0.95)500 \; ml = C_2(600 \; ml)$$
$$475 = C_2(600 \; ml)$$
$$\frac{475}{600} = C_2 = 0.792 = 79.2\%$$

Practice Set XI – 11   Solve.

1. The isopropyl alcohol on hand is 100%, but the desired strength is 70%. How much of the 100% stock solution is needed to make 2 gallons of 70% solution?

2. 36% HCl needs to be diluted to 1%. There is 100 ml of HCl on hand. How much will this make?

3. Make 15 L of a 10% formalin solution from a 100% stock solution. How much of the stock solution is needed? How much water is needed?

4. From a 10% formalin solution, prepare 20 L of: **a.** 5% solution   **b.** 1% solution

5. Determine the concentration of solution made from 1 Liter of 95% alcohol diluted with 150 ml of water.

6. A stock solution of sodium chloride is 9%. From it, prepare 5 L of a 0.9% saline solution.

7. Hydrochloric acid comes in a 90% stock solution. Using 50 ml of the acid and 40 ml of water, prepare a solution and determine its concentration.

8. Using 350 ml of 4% sulfuric acid and 200 ml of water, determine the concentration of the resultant diluted solution (round answer to nearest tenth of percent).

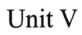
Unit V

Chapter 12
Statistics

In every technical occupation, an understanding of basic statistical concepts is essential. In this section, we explore some of the common statistical concepts, terms, numerical methods, and techniques that will form a basis for understanding. This is meant as an overview and in no way can this one chapter alone provide the technician with the skills they will surely need in a laboratory or clinical setting. A semester course in basic statistics is strongly recommended.

Knowledge of statistics allows you to make educated, informed decisions based upon data (information). Statistics is the study of collecting, organizing, and interpreting numerical information and making decisions based upon that information. Knowledge of statistics can help one make decisions about hospital occupancy rates, staffing issues, inventory and payroll.

In this chapter, the concepts of measures of central tendency and measures of variation will be explored.

In statistics there are three common "averages". The *mean*, denoted $\bar{x}$ (x–bar), which is the "average" most people think of when they think of the term average. The mean is arrived at by adding all the relevant items and dividing by how many of those items there are.

Example: Determine the mean of the following values. 85, 90, 92, 95, 94

$$\frac{85 + 90 + 92 + 95 + 94}{5} = 91.2 \qquad \text{The mean is 91.2}$$

Another type of average is called the *median*. Often, this number is more meaningful than the mean. The median is the middle number of a set of data that has been put in order from least to greatest. For the number set above, 85, 90, 92, 94, 95 . The median is 92. If the number of data values is even, then the median is the mean of the two middle values.

A third type of average is called the *mode*. The mode is the number that occurs most often in a set of data. For the previous values: 85, 90, 92, 94, 95, there is no number that occurs more than any other, therefore, there is no mode. For the values: 2, 3, 4, 4, 4, 5, 6, 6, 8, the mode is 4, since there are more representations of the value 4 than any other value.

These averages, called *measures of central tendency* describe some central point or measure of the data and indicate how data is grouped.

Measures of variation, on the other hand, describe how data is spread out. The *range* is a measure of the difference between the highest data value and the lowest. The measures of *variation* and *standard deviation* tell how much data varies around some middle value.

These measures of variation can describe if the data is all closely grouped or spread widely apart. *Standard deviation* is the square root of the *variance*. Many modern calculators perform these statistical functions making it easy to grasp the importance of the data rather than distracting you with tedious computations.

All fields have their own language and notation. Statistics is no different. Some notations typically found in the study of statistics include:

n used for the number of data values

$\bar{x}$ read as x-bar; symbolizes the mean

$\tilde{x}$ read as x-tilde; symbolizes the median

s^2 symbolizes the variance of a sample

s sample standard deviation; $s = \sqrt{s^2}$ standard deviation $= \sqrt{\text{variance}}$

Σ sigma (uppercase); summation = "to sum"

Summation notation is used in many statistical formulas. It is a notational device indicating addition and tells the user what should be added and the conditions for the addition.

These are called index numbers; the lower tells where to begin (in this case with the first data value) and the upper tells where to stop (the nth value)

$$\sum_{i=1}^{n} x_i$$

This part tells what is being added and what to do with it; do this part first, then add all the resultant values

In statistics, the index numbers are usually omitted since *all* the data values are used.

Examples: (i) Given the data: {2, 3, 6, 7, 9, 9}; Determine $\sum x$

This notation tells us to take each value in the data set, and then add, or sum, the result.

$$\sum x = 2 + 3 + 6 + 7 + 9 + 9 = 36$$

(ii) Given {2, 3, 6, 7, 9, 9}; Determine $\sum x^2$

$$\sum x^2 = 2^2 + 3^2 + 6^2 + 7^2 + 9^2 + 9^2 = 260$$

Note: in this case, first square each value, **then** add.

(iii) Given {2, 3, 6, 7, 9, 9}; Determine $\left(\sum x\right)^2$

$$\left(\sum x\right)^2 = \left(2 + 3 + 6 + 7 + 9 + 9\right)^2 = \left(36\right)^2 = 1296$$

Note the difference. In this case, the notation tells us to add the values **first**, then square the result.

Pay particular attention to the distinction between the second and third examples!

Practice Set XII – 1

Given the set of numbers $\{4, 8, 9, 2, 5\}$, Compute.

1. $\sum x$

2. $\dfrac{\sum x}{n}$

3. $\sum x^2$

4. $\sum (x - 5.6)$

5. $\sum (x - 5.6)^2$

Given the values $x_1 = 12, x_2 = 11, x_3 = 14, x_4 = 13$, Compute.

6. $\sum x$

7. $\sum x^2$

8. $\sum (x - 1)^2$

Now that you have had a little practice with using summation notation, we are going to introduce some formulas to use in computing statistics. Recall the mean, $\bar{x} = \dfrac{\sum x}{n}$, is the typical average which is the sum of all the data values divided by the number of pieces of data. The median, $\tilde{x}$, is the middle value of the ordered set of data. The mode is the data value that occurs more than any other number. If there is no such number, there is no mode. The range is the difference between the highest and lowest values. The variance, s^2, which is one measure of how data varies, is determined by the computational formula, $\text{variance} = \dfrac{n\sum x^2 - \left(\sum x\right)^2}{n(n-1)}$. The standard deviation, s, is the square root of the variance, $s = \sqrt{\text{variance}}$. We'll begin with a set of data, say test scores, and explore several important statistical concepts along the way.

Example: On 24 randomly chosen days, the number of patients visiting a clinic was recorded. Determine the mean, median, mode, range, variance and standard deviation for the data.

| 66 | 79 | 53 | 65 | 89 | 76 | 73 | 84 | 76 | 69 | 77 | 97 |
| 75 | 78 | 80 | 71 | 86 | 68 | 64 | 76 | 86 | 72 | 76 | 68 |

Order the scores from the smallest value to the largest. This is necessary to find the median.

53	69	76	80
64	71	76	84
65	72	76	86
66	73	77	86
68	75	78	89
68	76	79	97

With statistical problems, it is often helpful to organize the data in tables or columns. Since we need to know the sum of all the x and the sum of each of the x squared ...

x	x²
53	2809
64	4096
65	4225
66	4356
68	4624
68	4624
69	4761
71	5041
72	5184
73	5329
75	5625
76	5776
76	5776
76	5776
76	5776
77	5929
78	6084
79	6241
80	6400
84	7056
86	7396
86	7396
89	7921
97	9409
1804	137610	*Totals*

The number of data values, $n = 24$. The mean, $\bar{x} = \dfrac{\sum x}{n}$, $\dfrac{1804}{24} = 75.2$.

The median is the mean of the two middle numbers – the first and second values of 76 are the middle numbers – their mean is 76, so the median is 76.

The mode, the number that occurs most often is 76.

The range, the difference between the highest and lowest values, is 44 $(97 - 53 = 44)$.

The variance, found by formula, variance $= \dfrac{n\sum x^2 - \left(\sum x\right)^2}{n(n-1)}$

$$= \dfrac{(24)(137,610) - \left(1804\right)^2}{24(24-1)}$$

The substitutions for $n = 24$, the sum of the x's squared $= 137610$ and the sum of the x values $= 1804$. Simplify.

$$= \dfrac{3302640 - 3254416}{24 \times 23}$$

$$= \dfrac{48224}{552}$$

$$= 87.36 \quad \text{variance}$$

The standard deviation is the square root of the variance, $\sqrt{87.36} = 9.35$.

mean: $\bar{x} = 75.2$ median: $\tilde{x} = 76$ mode: 76

range: 44   variance: $s^2 = 87.36$ standard deviation: $s = 9.35$

A quick and easy way to organize and present data is to use a *stem–and–leaf diagram.*

A stem-and-leaf diagram has *stems* on the left of the vertical bar and *leaves* on the right. Since the data are all two-digits, the stems are the tens place while the units will be the leaves.

Key: 5 | 3 = 53

```
5 | 3
6 | 4 5 6 8 8 9
7 | 1 2 3 5 6 6 6 6 7 8 9
8 | 0 4 6 6 9
9 | 7
```

This diagram preserves all the original data and is easy to complete. On the other hand, it is not very useful for very large data sets.

Practice Set XII – 2

      Circle the correct response: **T – True   F – False**

1. For the data set: 5, 9, 12, 11, 2, 4, 9, and 8, the range would be 10.   T   F

2. For the sample: 1, 8, 7, 2, 9, 15, and 18, the mean is 7.6.   T   F

3. For the sample: 19, 21, 19, 17, 18, 19, and 21, the mode is 19.   T   F

4. For the sample: 1.3, 2.7, 8.9, 7.3, 9.2, and 8.1, the median is 8.9.   T   F

      Multiple Choice: Circle the letter of the correct response

5. Measures of central tendency are quantities which:

    (a) numerically describe data.   (b) describe the distribution of data.

    (c) describe the grouping of data.   (d) describe qualitative data.

6. Measures that describe how the data is distributed or spread out are:

    (a) range.   (b) variance.

    (c) standard deviation.   (d) all of the above.

7. Calculate the range and standard deviation (listed in that order) of the following sample test grades:

         87   75   68   57   69   78

    (a) 30, 9.3   (b) 30, 10.19   (c) 25, 9.3   (d) 25, 10.19

Practice Set XII – 3

1. Determine the mean and standard deviation for the temperatures taken from 10 readings.

100°F	101.7°F	99.9°F	103.2°F	102.4°F
100.5°F	102°F	104.5°F	102.8°F	103.5°F

2. Room occupancy rates often dictate how easy it might be to reserve a space for an outpatient procedure at the last minute and determine the average cost of that space. Occupancy rates for a clinic in a major city are given below.

56	89	79	71	70	60	60	61	62	63	64	65
81	73	68	72	56	59	60	62	73	64	72	67

a. Make a stem-and-leaf plot for the given data.

b. Determine the mean, median and mode.

c. Find the range and standard deviation.

3. The standard weight of an adolescent male is about 60 kilograms. Determine the mean, median and mode of the weights of the males treated in a certain practice. Also find the range, variance and standard deviation. Weights given in kg.

58   60   62   64   61   56   62   62   54   64

4. There is concern about staff turnover in a particular practice. A survey was conducted and the number of months that staff was on the job was recorded. Find the mean, median, mode, range and standard deviation for the number of months that employees have been on the job.

10   2   40   15   27   6   9   8   4   25   30
38   14   5   12   18   20   35   44   7   24   9

The *weighted average* is a measure of the mean which assigns certain "weights" to different measures. For example, in a particular class, term papers may account for 20% of your grade, quizzes for 30%, tests for 40%, attendance for 10%. Your grade for each item is affected by the weight of that item. The formula, $\bar{x}_w = \dfrac{\sum xw}{\sum w}$, uses each value for *x* multiplied by its weight and the result summed, then divided by the sum of the weights.

Example: Sally and Bill were in the same English class. Sally had grade averages of 90 for papers, 89 for tests, 95 for quizzes and 100 for attendance. Bill had grade averages of 84 for papers, 93 for tests, 86 for quizzes and 85 for attendance. Determine the weighted average of each student.

$$\frac{90(.20)+89(.40)+95(.30)+100(.10)}{.20+.30+.40+.10}$$ Add the grades multiplied by their corresponding weights

Add the weights

$$\frac{18+35.6+28.5+10}{1} = 92.1$$ Simplify. Sally's grade is a 92

$$\frac{84(.20)+93(.40)+86(.30)+85(.10)}{.20+.30+.40+.10}$$ Add the grades multiplied by their corresponding weights

Add the weights

$$\frac{16.8+37.2+25.8+8.5}{1} = 88.3$$ Simplify. Bill's grade is an 88

5. A pay scale is determined by scores given to an employee by their supervisor for such things as accurate records, good work habits, attitude dealing with customers and ability to get along with fellow employees. Weights are assigned as follows: 2 for attendance and good work habits, 3 for record keeping, 4 for customer relations and 2 for interaction with coworkers. What would be an employee's weighted average if her scores were, on a scale from 1 to 10, 9 for attendance, 8 for keeping accurate records, 8 for customer relations, and 6 for getting along with coworkers.

6. Anna and Bonita were in the same literature class. Grades were determined on a weighted scale according to the following: tests accounted for 35% of the grade, quizzes 20%, term papers were 25% and the final exam was worth 20% of the grade. Anna had test average of 90, quiz average of 80, 93 on her papers and she scored 88 on the final.

Bonita had an 84 average on her tests, a 92 average on quizzes, an 89 average for her papers and she did very well on the final exam scoring a 95.

Determine the grade, rounded to the nearest whole number, for each of the girls.

Selected Solutions

Chapter 1

Practice Set I – 1

1. 20   **3.** 64   **5.** 99   **7.** 448   **9.** 3333   **11.** 4   **13.** 3   **15.** 57   **17.** 32   **19.** MCMLXXIII

21. IX   **23.** XXIX   **25.** XLIX   **27.** MMCCXXII   **29.** IV   **31.** LIV   **33.** LXXVI

Chapter 2

Practice Set II - 1

1. a. $\dfrac{2}{4}$ **b.** $\dfrac{3}{8}$ **c.** $\dfrac{5}{9}$ **d.** $\dfrac{5}{12}$ **3. a.** $\dfrac{1}{36}$ yard   **b.** $\dfrac{35}{36}$ yd   **c.** $\dfrac{13}{36}$ yd   **d.** $\dfrac{19}{36}$ yd

5. a. $\$\dfrac{12}{100}$ **b.** $\$\dfrac{37}{100}$ **c.** $\$\dfrac{50}{100}$ **d.** $\$\dfrac{99}{100}$

Practice Set II-2

1. $\dfrac{3}{5}$ **3.** $\dfrac{1}{2}$ **5.** 4   **7.** $\dfrac{1}{2}$ **9.** $\dfrac{8}{9}$ **11.** $\dfrac{5}{9}$

Practice Set II - 3

1. $3\dfrac{1}{3}$ **3.** $6\dfrac{1}{4}$ **5.** $2\dfrac{3}{16}$ **7.** $\dfrac{13}{3}$ **9.** $\dfrac{19}{10}$ **11.** $\dfrac{35}{9}$

Practice Set II - 4

1. a. $\dfrac{1}{4}$ **b.** $\dfrac{1}{6}$ **c.** $\dfrac{24}{25}$ **d.** $\dfrac{1}{4}$ **e.** $\dfrac{1}{2}$ **f.** $\dfrac{1}{6}$ **g.** $\dfrac{1}{8}$ **h.** $\dfrac{1}{9}$

3. a. 3   **b.** $6\dfrac{6}{7}$ **c.** $6\dfrac{1}{9}$ **d.** $7\dfrac{1}{9}$ **e.** $21\dfrac{1}{4}$ **f.** $3\dfrac{4}{7}$ **g.** $4\dfrac{1}{5}$ **h.** $5\dfrac{1}{4}$

Chapter 3

Practice Set III – 1

1. $\dfrac{4}{3}=1\dfrac{1}{3}$ **3.** $\dfrac{7}{2}=3\dfrac{1}{2}$ **5.** $\dfrac{20}{7}=2\dfrac{6}{7}$ **7.** $\dfrac{5}{3}=1\dfrac{2}{3}$

Practice Set III – 2

1. $\dfrac{1}{9}$ **3.** $\dfrac{1}{12}$ **5.** $\dfrac{6}{20}=\dfrac{3}{10}$ **7.** $\dfrac{15}{32}$

Practice Set III – 3

1. $\frac{4}{15}$ 3. $\frac{3}{20}$ 5. $\frac{3}{5}$ 7. $\frac{1}{4}$ 9. $\frac{1}{6}$ 11. $\frac{2}{5}$

Practice Set III – 4

1. 32   3. 22   5. $13\frac{1}{5}$ 7. $9\frac{1}{3}$ 9. $9\frac{4}{5}$ 11. $56\frac{1}{4}$ 13. $8\frac{5}{16}$

Practice Set III – 5

1. $41\frac{1}{4}$ 3. 21 pounds

Practice Set III – 6

1. $\frac{5}{6}$ 3. $1\frac{1}{5}$ 5. $\frac{5}{9}$ 7. $2\frac{1}{10}$ 9. 48

Practice Set III – 7

1. 15   3. 16   5. $13\frac{1}{2}$ 7. $106\frac{2}{3}$ 9. 210

Practice Set III – 8

1. $\frac{7}{40}$ 3. $\frac{1}{16}$ 5. $\frac{3}{11}$

Practice Set III – 9

1. $26\frac{2}{3}$ 3. $\frac{13}{30}$ 5. $\frac{1}{4}$ 7. 18   9. $1\frac{1}{5}$

Practice Set III – 10

1. $\frac{7}{9}$ 3. $\frac{2}{5}$ 5. $\frac{1}{2}$ 7. $\frac{1}{6}$ 9. $1\frac{1}{2}$ 11. $1\frac{1}{2}$

13. $5\frac{1}{3}$ 15. 12   17. 8   19. 16   21. 24   23. $\frac{1}{4}$

25. $\frac{10}{29}$ 27. 8   29. $\frac{8}{25}$ 31. 6   33. 1

Chapter 4

Practice Set IV – 1

1. $\dfrac{7}{8}$ 3. $\dfrac{4}{5}$ 5. $\dfrac{3}{7}$ 7. $\dfrac{5}{4} = 1\dfrac{1}{4}$

Practice Set IV – 2

1. $\dfrac{1}{3}$ 3. $\dfrac{2}{3}$ 5. $\dfrac{2}{3}$ 7. $\dfrac{5}{8}$ 9. $\dfrac{3}{8}$ 11. $\dfrac{9}{14}$

13. $\dfrac{1}{3}$ 15. $1\dfrac{5}{8}$

Practice Set IV – 3

1. $13\dfrac{5}{12}$ 3. $19\dfrac{5}{8}$ 5. $15\dfrac{3}{4}$ 7. $22\dfrac{3}{5}$ 9. $13\dfrac{1}{2}$ 11. $15\dfrac{1}{2}$

13. $16\dfrac{1}{2}$ 15. $8\dfrac{7}{9}$

Practice Set IV – 4

1. $3\dfrac{11}{16}$ 3. $4\dfrac{17}{20}$

Practice Set IV – 5

1. $3\dfrac{11}{12}$ 3. $8\dfrac{2}{3}$

Practice Set IV – 6

1. $\dfrac{1}{3}$ 3. $\dfrac{7}{11}$

Practice Set IV – 7

1. $\dfrac{3}{8}$ 3. $\dfrac{1}{6}$ 5. $\dfrac{7}{32}$ 7. $\dfrac{7}{20}$ 9. $\dfrac{3}{5}$ 11. 1

Practice Set IV – 8

1. $3\frac{3}{8}$ **3.** $4\frac{1}{4}$ **5.** $1\frac{1}{6}$ **7.** $9\frac{1}{12}$ **9.** $3\frac{7}{15}$

Practice Set IV – 9

1. $\frac{11}{15}$ **3.** $1\frac{1}{2}$ **5.** $1\frac{21}{22}$ **7.** $7\frac{1}{5}$ **9.** $\frac{13}{20}$

Practice Set IV – 10

1. $\frac{1}{9}$ **3.** $\frac{1}{20}$ **5.** $\frac{49}{18} = 2\frac{13}{18}$

Practice Set IV – Chapter Review

1. $\frac{15}{17}$ **3.** $1\frac{11}{16}$ **5.** $\frac{3}{20}$ **7.** $12\frac{43}{60}$ **9.** $1\frac{71}{72}$ **11.** 1

13. $7\frac{31}{60}$ **15.** $\frac{23}{24}$ **17.** $1\frac{1}{6}$ **19.** $4\frac{11}{14}$ **21.** $19\frac{11}{12}$ **23.** 0

Chapter 5

Practice Set V – 1

1. 0.9   **3.** 0.25   **5.** 0.012   **7.** 0.5'

Practice Set V – 2

1. 0.171875   **3.** 0.625   **5.** 0.25   **7.** 0.078125   **9.** 1.375
11. 0.75   **13.** 2.625   **15.** 1.140625

Practice Set V – 3

1. $\frac{3}{50}$ **3.** $\frac{99}{200}$ **5.** $\frac{63}{100}$ **7.** $\frac{3}{10}$ **9.** $1\frac{47}{250}$

Practice Set V – 4

    1. 0.873   **3.** 0.778   **5.** 0 .621   **7.** 0.65   **9.** 0.37   **11.** 0.43
    13. 590   **15.** 1760   **17.** 1600   **19.** 1910   **21.** 1070   **23.** 50
    25. 1430   **27.** 876900

Practice Set V – 5

    1. 25.108   **3.** 11.2615   **5.** 3.605   **7.** 22.506   **9.** 0.0883
    11. 17.73   **13.** 2.8

Practice Set V – 6

    1. 91.75   **3.** 10,998.92   **5.** 9.2869   **7.** 0.0242

Chapter 6

Practice Set VI – 1

    1. 1.40   **3.** 0.1414   **5.** 0.049764

Practice Set VI – 2

    1. 105   **3.** 0.3216   **5.** 2388.33   **7.** 0.0066091   **9.** 800.46873
    11. $148.48   **13.** $576.24   **15.** $27.90

Practice Set VI – 3

    1. 36   **3.** 47   **5.** 2450

Practice Set VI – 4

    1. 0.26   **3.** 0.058   **5.** 0.22   **7.** 3.01   **9.** 2.05

Practice Set VI – 5

    1. 30   **3.** 150   **5.** 80

Practice Set VI – 6

1. 10891   **3.** 32.4   **5.** 64   **7.** 383.4   **9.** 100,100
11. 80   **13.** 67.6

Practice Set VI – 7

1. 0.343   **3.** 34.3   **5.** 343   **7.** 3430   **9.** 3.43
11. 0.0343   **13.** 34300   **15.** 3.43   **17.** 0.00343

Practice Set VI – 8 Review

1. 0.9828   **3.** 23.814   **5.** 39.6381   **7.** 1.2288   **9.** 2.02608
11. 0.13792   **13.** 10.76154   **15.** 15.65541   **17.** 13.08335   **19.** 5.74875
21. 5.25   **23.** 18.48   **25.** 60.7087   **27.** 1078   **29.** 1.4887
31. 0.0171

1. 900   **3.** 2   **5.** 2.920   **7.** 0.041   **9.** 100.5
11. 9   **13.** 5   **15.** 20.2   **17.** 0.426   **19.** 0.098
21. 835.9   **23.** 540

Practice Set VI – 9

1. 31,420   **3.** 31.42   **5.** 0.3142   **7.** 0.03142   **9.** 0.003142

Practice Set VI – 10

1. 2310; 23.1   **3.** 48,236; 0.048236   **5.** 469.1; 0.04691
7. 0.08569; 8,569,000   **9.** 187.54; 1.8754

Practice Set VI – 11

In general, there is no real difference between 1×10^7 and 10^7. Either should be acceptable.

1. 1×10^5 **3.** 1×10^6 **5.** 1×10^{-2} **7.** 1×10^{-10} **9.** 1×10^3
11. 1,000,000   **13.** 1000   **15.** 0.001
17. 0.01   **19.** 100

Practice Set VI – 12

1. 20,000   **3.** 0.0033   **5.** 0.0000000847   **7.** 8.39×10^{-4} **9.** 8,769,000,000
11. 0.0000006798   **13.** 3.57×10^{-3} **15.** 0.0000075 **17.** 40,000,000
19. 4.5789×10^{4} **21.** 8.32467×10^{3} **23.** 3.57×10^{-3} **25.** 1.0×10^{-5}

Fraction Review

1. $3\frac{25}{27}$ **3.** $20\frac{1}{12}$ **5.** $2\frac{21}{40}$ **7.** $3\frac{1}{5}$ **9.** $1\frac{1}{12}$

11. $9\frac{1}{3}$ **13.** $4\frac{3}{4}$ **15.** $3\frac{1}{2}$ **17.** $10\frac{1}{4}$ **19.** $\frac{7}{45}$

21. $\frac{66}{125}$ **23.** $16\frac{4}{5}$ **25.** $\frac{5}{18}$ **27.** $\frac{3}{10}$ **29.** $\frac{9}{10}$

31. $\frac{1}{2}$ **33.** $812\frac{1}{2}$ **35.** $3\frac{1}{5}$ **37.** $\frac{3}{10}$ **39.** $\frac{3}{10}$

41. $8\frac{1}{4}$ **43.** $\frac{3}{4}$ **45.** $\frac{4}{21}$ **47.** $3\frac{9}{31}$ **49.** $\frac{1}{2}$

51. $1\frac{13}{29}$

Chapter 7

Practice Set VII – 1
1. 0.15   **3.** 0.943   **5.** 0.09   **7.** 0.4   **9.** 0.05

Practice Set VII – 2
1. 10%   **3.** 90%   **5.** 76.2%   **7.** 12.5%   **9.** 8.5%   **11.** 225%

Practice Set VII – 3
1. $\frac{3}{5}$ **3.** $\frac{11}{10} = 1\frac{1}{10}$ **5.** $\frac{2}{25}$

Practice Set VII – 4
1. 25%   **3.** 83.3%   **5.** 18.8%   **7.** 70%

Practice Set VII – 5

1. 0.125　　**3.** 0.5711　　**5.** 0.095　　**7.** 33%　　**9.** 98.7%　　**11.** 11%

13. 12.5%　　**15.** 14.3%　　**17.** 11.1%　　**19.** 9.1%　　**21.** $\dfrac{1}{50}$　　**23.** $\dfrac{1}{5}$

25. $\dfrac{8}{25}$　　**27.** $\dfrac{77}{200}$

	Fraction	Decimal	Percent
29.	$\dfrac{2}{25}$	0.08	8%
31.	$\dfrac{37}{40}$	0.925	92.5%
33.	$\dfrac{3}{7}$	0.429	42.9%
35.	650	650.00	65,000%
37.	$1\dfrac{1}{4}$	1.25	125%
39.	$\dfrac{333}{1000}$	0.333	33.3%
41.	$1\dfrac{5}{9}$	1.556	155.6%

Practice Set VII – 6

1. 50　　**3.** 500　　**5.** 50　　**7.** 75　　**9.** 300　　**11.** 30.006

Practice Set VII – 7

1. $705　　**3.** $465.80

Practice Set VII – 8

1. 29.6%　　**3.** 10%　　**5.** 15.6%　　**7.** 8.1%　　**9.** 70.8%

Practice Set VII – 9

    1. $5.83   **3.** $5.28   **5.** $7.75

Practice Set VII – 10

    1. 4.48   **3.** 160   **5.** 112.7   **7.** 0.03   **9.** 307.5 sq ft; 1537.5 sq ft

Practice Set VII – 11

Item	Company A list price	Company A new price	Company B list price	Company B new price
general operating scissors	$6.10	**$4.76**	$4.45	**$4.78**
iris scissors	$7.05	**$5.50**	$5.00	**$5.38**
surgical cotton wadding	$4.20	**$3.28**	$3.85	**$4.14**
Needle holders	$4.25	**$3.32**	$3.00	**$3.23**
Endotracheal tubes	$2.38	**$1.86**	$1.93	**$2.07**

Practice Set VII – 12

Either g% or $\frac{g}{dl}$ is acceptable.

1. 14 g% or 14 $\frac{g}{dl}$ **3.** 0.5 g%   **5.** 4 g%   **7.** 0.4 mg%

9. 5%   **11.** 10%   **13.** 70%

Chapter 8

Practice Set VIII – 1

    1. 80:40 = 2:1   **3.** 12:5

Practice Set VIII – 2

1. $\dfrac{1}{3} = 0.33$ 3. $\dfrac{1}{3} = 0.33$ 5. $\dfrac{1}{8} = 0.125 = 0.13$

Practice Set VIII – 3

1. $\dfrac{5\ g}{100\ ml} = \dfrac{1\ g}{20\ ml}$ 3. $\dfrac{100\ mg}{1\ cc}$ 5. $\dfrac{25\ mg}{1\ ml}$ 7. $\dfrac{1\ cc}{5\ lbs}$

Practice Set VIII – 4

1. 20   3. 1.5   5. 40   7. 1000   9. 9   11. 0.4

13. 400   15. 0.01 or $\dfrac{1}{100}$ 17. $171

Practice Set VIII – 5

1. 30 ml   3. 0.4 cc

Chapter 8 Review

1. 1   3. 1   5. 1.125   7. 27   9. 1.5   11. 100
13. 10.769   15. 27   17. 15   19. 7 cc   21. 13 cc   22. 1.875 mg
23. 7 drops   25. 5.5 ml   27. 2.32 cc   29. 9 g   31. 17 mg   33. 2.75 mg
35. 20 g   37. 300 cc   39. 4.8 drops   41. 3.5 mg   43. 32 mg   45. 50 mg
47. 5 cc   49. 0.52 ml   51. 0.9 ml   53. 0.36 cc   54. 3.25 mg   55. 4.2 cc
57. 0.4 ml

Chapter 9

Practice Set IX – 1

1. meniscus   3. 1 g/cc   5. 10.5

Practice Set IX – 2

1. hecto   3. none   5. milli   7. centi

Practice Set IX – 3

1. dm; $^1/_{10}$ meters   **3.** dkg; 10 grams   **5.** dl; $^1/_{10}$ liters   **7.** g; 1 gram

9. dg; $^1/_{10}$ g   **11.** L; 1 liter   **13.** hl; 100 L   **15.** ml; $^1/_{1000}$ L

Practice Set IX – 4

1. 1200   **3.** 2100   **5.** 5510   **7.** 3000

9. 5,151,200   **11.** 0.112   **13.** 0.0123   **15.** 0.0235

17. 0.0034   **19.** 0.1511235

Practice Set IX – 5

1. pt   **3.** c   **5.** teaspoon   **7.** ounce

9. oz   **11.** gal   **13.** in   **15.** gr

Practice Set IX – 6

1. 10   **3.** 18   **5.** 10   **7.** 27   **9.** 108

11. 1314   **13.** 10,560   **15.** 9

Practice Set IX – 7

1. 1   **3.** 8; 4; 1   **5.** 1   **7.** 72   **9.** 0.58

11. 1.5   **13.** $^1/_3$ **15.** 60   **17.** 384

Practice Set IX – 8

1. 7   **3.** 12.5   **5.** 2.85   **7.** 1.5   **9.** 45   **11.** 908

Practice Set IX – 9

1. 104°F   **3.** 98.6°F   **5.** 0°C   **7.** 113°F   **9.** 37.8°C   **11.** −17.8°C

13. −23.3°C   **15.** 77°F   **17.** −12.2°C

Practice Set IX – 10

1. 45	**3.** 2	**5.** 90	**7.** 1136.36	**9.** 592.5
11. 20	**13.** 3.55	**15.** 30	**17.** 1.5	**19.** 3.33

Practice Set IX – 11

1. 2	**3.** 2	**5.** 40	**7.** $1^2/_3$	**9.** 6	**11.** 6.67
13. 1	**15.** 0.67	**17.** 1.06	**19.** 2.11	**21.** 12.68	**23.** 0.21
25. 3	**27.** 3.25	**29.** 2.4	**31.** 0.8	**33.** 1.59	**35.** 150

Practice Set IX – 12

1. 0.05	**3.** 1; 0.5; 473	**5.** 0.5	**7.** 250	**9.** 30
11. 15	**13.** 1	**15.** 180	**17.** 0.15	**19.** 4; 8; 3785
21. 500	**22.** 0.6	**23.** 0.25	**25.** 1500	**27.** 1
29. 30	**31.** 2			

Chapter 10

Practice Set X – 1

1. 8	**3.** 7	**5.** 54	**7.** 120	**9.** 19	**11.** 10	**13.** 7

Practice Set X – 2

1. 25   **3.** $4\frac{5}{8}$ **5.** 19   **7.** 144

Practice Set X – 3

1. 29   **3.** $-3\frac{1}{2}$ **5.** 98   **7.** –8.5   **9.** –1   **11.** $5\frac{1}{2}$ **13.** 11.5   **15.** 78

Practice Set X – 4

1. −11 **3.** $\dfrac{6}{17}$ **5.** $-20\dfrac{1}{2}$ **7.** $2\dfrac{3}{7}$ **9.** $7\dfrac{2}{3}$

Practice Set X – 5

1. $x \geq 18$ **3.** $x > 7$ **5.** $x < 7\dfrac{6}{7}$ **7.** $x > 32$ **9.** $x \geq 7$

Practice Set X – 6

1. $x > 5$ **3.** $x < 1\dfrac{1}{3}$ **5.** $x > 11.5$ **7.** $x < -3$ **9.** $x < \dfrac{5}{8}$ **11.** $x \geq -\dfrac{4}{5}$

Applications

1. $25 + .10m = 35 + .08m$
$.02m = 10$
$m = 500 \; miles$

If you drive 500 miles, which plan doesn't matter. For 720 miles, the first plan costs $97 and the other plan cost $92.60. Therefore, the $35 per day plan is less expensive.

3. No; No; 100ºF is not too high

5. 3 cc; 7 vials

Practice Set X – 7

1.

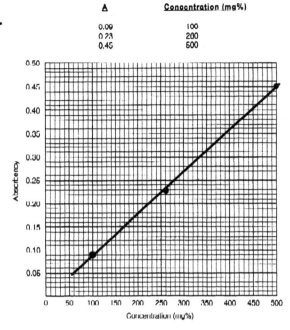

A	Concentration (mg%)
0.09	100
0.23	200
0.45	500

1. A. 175   **C.** 165   **E.** 130

2. A. 2%   **C.** 6%   **E.** 5.4%

3. A. (1, 1)   **C.** (3.4, 0)   **E.** (4.6, –1.2)   **G.** (6.6, –3)   **I.** (8, 2.2)
K. (6.1, 0.8)   **M.** (5.8, 2.4)

Chapter 11

Practice Set XI – 1

1. 400 mg   **3.a.** 900 mg   **b.** 204 mg   **5.** 20.83 cc

Practice Set XI – 2

1. 8.5 cc   **3.** 18.5 cc   **5.** 0.9 cc   **7.** 1800 mg and **b.** 859.1 mg
9. 144,000 units   **9.b.** 4 bags

Practice Set XI – 3

1.a. 4000 mg **b.** 2500 mg **3.a.** 2 – 450 mg capsules/day; 12 for 6 days
3.b. 2 – 150 mg tablets/day; 20 tablets for 10 days **5.** 25 mg = 1 – 25 mg tablet
7.a.i. 2280 mg **ii.** 2700 mg **b.** 2700 mg **9.** 42.5 units

Practice Set XI – 4

1. a. 8.0 cc **b.** 4.8 cc **c.** 3.2 cc

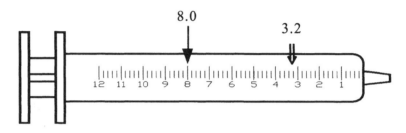

Practice Set XI – 5

1. 360 g **3.** 25 g **5.** 150 ml **7.** 6 g Iodine, 12 g potassium iodine
9. 2.25 g **11.** 1 g

Practice Set XI – 6

1. 22.5 g **3.** 32.5 ml **5.** 325 ml **7.** 0.25 g **9.** 20 g **11.** 95%
13. 2% **15.** 0.9%

Practice Set XI – 7

1. 5.34 mg **3.a.** 818.2 mg/dose; 24, 545.5 mg total
3.b. 1750 mg/dose; 21,000 mg total **c.** 1125 mg/dose; 18,000 mg total
d. 2272.7 mg/dose; 47,727.3 mg total **5.a.** 0.55 mg is 1.375 vials

Practice Set XI – 8

1. 1.75 L + 0.75 L of diluent
3. 2.4 L formalin + 9.6 L H_2O
5. 2000 ml of 1% + 1980 ml H_2O
7. 2.1 L of 100% + 0.9 L diluent

Practice Set XI – 9

1. 0.7 L or 700 ml of 100% needed and 0.3 L of diluent
3. 3000 ml (3 L) of 5% can be made using 2.5 L water
5. 5 L of 2% can be made by adding 4 L of diluent

Practice Set XI – 10

1. a. 1.5 L 100% stock + 28.5 L diluent   b. 0.3 L of 100% stock + 29.7 L diluent
3. a. 5.7 L of stock + 0.3 L diluent   b. 6.6 L stock + 2.4 L diluent
5. 2.1 gallons of 100% stock solution + 0.9 gal of diluent
7. 7200 ml can be made by diluting what is on hand with 7000 ml of H_2O.
9. a. 250 ml of 10% + 250 ml of diluent   b. 35 ml of 10% + 315 ml diluent

Practice Set XI – 11

1. 1.4 gal of 100% stock sol needed
3. 1.5 L of 100% stock + 13.5 L H_2O
5. 82.6%   7. 50%

Chapter 12

Practice Set XII – 1

1. 28   3. 190   5. 33.2   7. 630

Practice Set XII – 2

1. True   3. True   5. c   7. b

Practice Set XII – 3

1. $\bar{x} = 102.1°F$; $s^2 = 2.385$; $s = 1.54°F$

2. **a.** Stem and Leaf **Key** $5\,|\,6 = 56$

$$
\begin{array}{c|l}
8 & 1\ \ 9 \\
7 & 0\ \ 1\ \ 2\ \ 2\ \ 3\ \ 3\ \ 9 \\
6 & 0\ \ 0\ \ 0\ \ 1\ \ 2\ \ 2\ \ 3\ \ 4\ \ 4\ \ 5\ \ 7\ \ 8 \\
5 & 6\ \ 6\ \ 9
\end{array}
$$

c. Range = 33; variance = 67.30 and standard deviation = 8.2

3. mean $\bar{x} = 60.3\ kg$; median $\tilde{x} = 61.5\ kg$; mode = 62 kg; range = 10 kg; variance $s^2 = 11.2222$; standard deviation $s = 3.33$

5. $\bar{x}_w = \dfrac{\sum xw}{\sum w} = \dfrac{9(2) + 8(3) + 8(4) + 6(2)}{2 + 3 + 4 + 2} = \dfrac{86}{11} = 7.8$